FOOD is MEDICINE

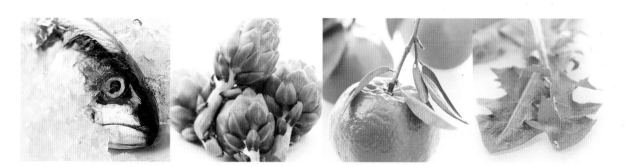

To Roberta, Emilie, and Etienne

Food is Medicine

Pierre Jean Cousin

Ths revised edition first published in the United Kingdom and Ireland in 2006 by

Duncan Baird Publishers Ltd

Sixth Floor, Castle House

75–76 Wells Street

London W1T 3QH

Conceived, created and designed by Duncan Baird Publishers

Managing designer: Manisha Patel

Design and photographic art direction: Steve Painter

DTP designer: Joy Wheeler

Editorial assistant: Jessica Hughes

Commissioned photography: William Lingwood

Stylists: Sunil Vijayakar and Helen Trent

British Library Cataloguing-in-Publication Data:

A catalogue record for this book is available from the British Library

10 9 8 7 6 5 4 3 2 1

ISBN 10: 1-84483-244-9

ISBN 13: 9-781844-832446

Typeset in Helvetica

Colour reproduction by Colourscan, Singapore

Printed in Singapore by Imago

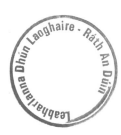

FOOD IS MEDICINE

The Practical Guide To Healing Foods

PIERRE JEAN COUSIN

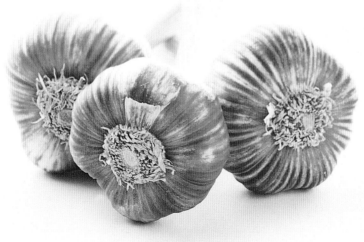

DUNCAN BAIRD PUBLISHERS

LONDON

contents

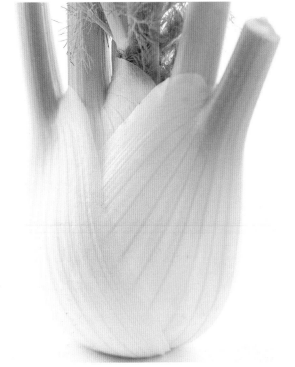

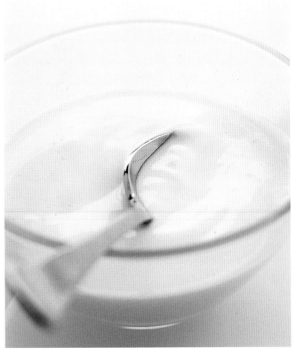

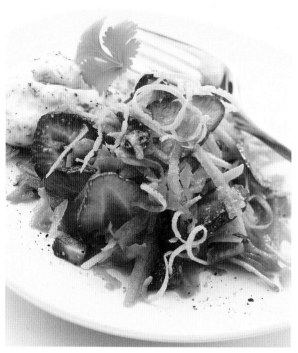

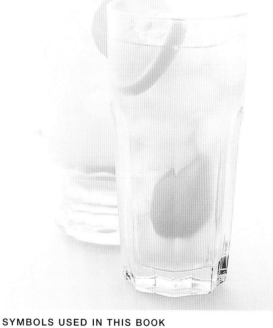

SYMBOLS USED IN THIS BOOK

★ IMPORTANT NUTRIENTS AND
    OTHER ACTIVE INGREDIENTS

● BODY SYSTEM AND AILMENT

! WARNING

✔ BENEFICIAL FOODS AND
    OTHER RECOMMENDATIONS

✗ FOODS, DRINKS AND
    PRACTICES TO AVOID

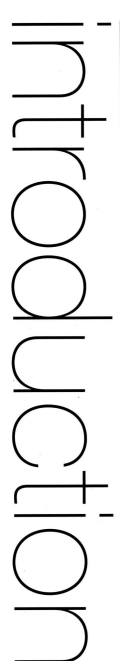

One of the most important ways in which we can influence our health is by monitoring what we eat. Eating unhealthily – too much animal fat, salt, sugar and artificial additives – can cause irreparable damage to our bodies, especially to the cardiovascular system and the kidneys. Eating healthily can increase vitality, immunity and life expectancy. We can also influence the health of future generations by teaching our children healthy eating habits.

Food can be used not only to prevent illness but also to treat it. Throughout the ages, and in all cultures, food has played an important role in healing the sick. Yet in contemporary Western societies the emphasis in healthcare has moved from traditional methods, such as diet, to modern medical techniques and a reliance on pharmaceuticals. As a result, self-help dietary remedies are rarely considered. As an experienced practitioner of a range of complementary therapies, I firmly believe in bringing the healing power of foods back to where it belongs – in our homes.

the principles of healthy eating

The mainstay of a healthy diet is plenty of unrefined complex carbohydrates and fibre. Foods such as beans, lentils, potatoes, wholemeal pasta, wholegrain bread and cereals should make up – quite literally – the bulk of our diet. Protein-rich foods, such as meat or fish, can be added to this carbohydrate base in small amounts. Contrary to popular belief, we don't need very much protein for good health and it is not necessary to eat meat, fish and dairy products as a daily source of protein. The other essential ingredients in a healthy diet are vitamins, minerals and phytochemicals (biologically-active substances in plants) which are found in abundance in fruit and vegetables, and essential fatty acids from nuts, seeds, oily fish and oils such as olive oil.

This basic template for healthy eating closely matches the traditional diet that is – or was – eaten in many cultures. Civilizations throughout history have relied upon a combination of cereals and pulses for their staple diet. In Asia this combination is rice and soya; in America corn and beans; in Europe wheat, rye, barley, oats or buckwheat and beans, lentils or other pulses; and in Africa it is wheat, millet or sorghum and beans or chickpeas. Traditionally, a variety of fruit and vegetables (often eaten raw) has complemented this diet, together with small amounts of meat and fish when available. Fermented foods, such as cheese, yoghurt, curd, fish sauce, pickled vegetables, cider, beer and wine – all of which have a beneficial effect on the intestine – also feature in the traditional diet. This diet is ideally suited to the human body – it is rich in friendly bacteria, fibre and nutrients and helps to maintain a healthy biological balance in the intestine.

It is very easy to adopt the healthy eating habits that are characteristic of such diets by following these simple common-sense measures:

● Buy more fresh fruit and vegetables (they are rich in antioxidants – substances that help to prevent degenerative disease such as cancer and heart disease), cereals, pulses and fish.
● Cut down on meat, dairy products and convenience foods.
● Replace meat with oily fish.
● Tailor food intake to match your actual calorie needs (for most people this means eating less).
● Buy a cook book that focuses on the Mediterranean diet.
● Reduce your intake of sugar, coffee, tea, fizzy drinks and alcohol.
● Eat at regular intervals (up to five times a day if this suits your needs).

- Eat food that is in season and, ideally, locally produced according to organic principles.
- Make sure that your diet is as varied as possible.
- Use fresh ingredients as often as possible; avoid canned or dried food which contains additives.
- Be flexible in your eating – aim for balance and enjoyment. Avoid rigid dietary programmes.

how the modern diet fails

These principles of healthy eating contrast starkly with modern Western eating habits. Whereas the diet of our pre-industrial ancestors was rich in fresh produce, the modern diet, which has evolved over the last 50–60 years, is characterized by food that contains preservatives, colorants, taste enhancers, sugar, caffeine and even traces of fertilizers, pesticides, antibiotics, hormones and metals. This leads to a proliferation of unhealthy bacteria in the gut, an accumulation of toxins in the body, poor digestion and an increased likelihood of allergies, cardiovascular disease and a range of cancers, including breast and bowel cancer.

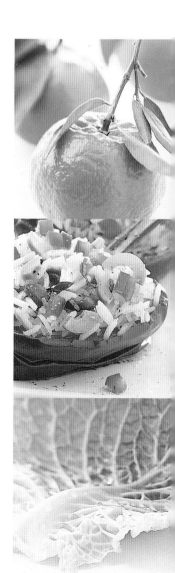

In the West, food is abundant (the amount produced far exceeds our needs) and relatively cheap owing to modern production and processing techniques. These techniques have created what has been termed "food industrialization" – the production of large amounts of food quickly and cheaply at the expense of quality and nutritional content. Paradoxically, although we now have more choice in what we can eat, less time is devoted to the selection, preparation and consumption of food. Our diets often consist of a limited number of ingredients that we continue eating out of routine and convenience.

Much of the food that we buy is impoverished. For example, when fresh produce is out of season in one country, it is often imported from another, and much of its vitamin content is lost during transit or storage in refrigerators or on supermarket shelves.

Goodness is also depleted in the process of sterilization: in order to make fresh food "safe" and prolong shelf-life by eliminating micro-organisms, it is often sterilized or irradiated – yet this procedure renders it, quite literally, lifeless. Although all unhealthy, disease-causing bacteria are killed in the process, all the "good" bacteria and ferments are also destroyed. These are important for digestion and in maintaining a healthy and balanced environment in the intestine. Most milk, for example, is pasteurized, with the result that it does not contain natural ferments and is difficult for many people to break down and digest. Milk products that have not been pasteurized, such as live yoghurt (which is full of lactobacilli bacteria), are well tolerated by most people. Another consequence of sterilization is that, if food is left out of the refrigerator for too long or is reheated too many times, micro-organisms, such as listeria, will re-establish themselves. Without competition from good bacteria, unhealthy ones can proliferate unchecked and cause disease.

Industrialized food production is partly responsible for a range of contemporary health problems, such as male hormone imbalance (linked to the misuse of hormones in animals), the advent of antibiotic-resistant strains of bacteria (linked to the routine addition of antibiotics to animal feed), salmonella in poultry and eggs (linked to poor living conditions among animals), and Creutzfeldt-Jacob disease (linked to bovine spongiform encephalopathy or BSE, a disease affecting cows that is caused by contaminated cattle feed). Genetic modification of food is the

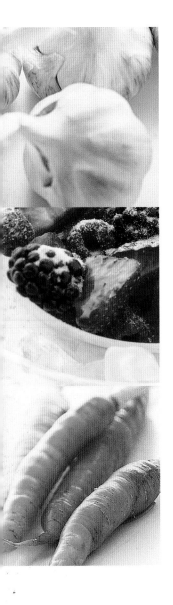

latest in a catalogue of food-production experiments that I believe may have harmful, long-term effects on human health and the environment. The defensive attitude of scientists who argue that "no evidence exists that genetically-modified (GM) food is unsafe" needs to be challenged – this kind of negative statement does not constitute proof that GM food is safe.

Owing to the wide-ranging effects of food industrialization it is important that, as consumers, we make informed choices about what we buy – not just favouring foods that are unprocessed and grown according to organic principles, but also excluding products that are nutritionally empty and preserved and enhanced in artificial ways.

the medicinal value of food

Our knowledge of the healing power of food is based upon thousands of years of tradition and empirical observation. Modern scientific research now confirms the curative abilities of certain compounds contained in foods that have been used therapeutically through the ages. For example, the potent antibacterial action of allicin, a substance found in garlic, is well documented. So too are the protective and healing properties of antioxidants and essential oils found in fruit, vegetables, herbs and spices. Some pharmacologically-active ingredients are extracted from food and sold in tablet form. Cynarin, for example, is an active ingredient that is extracted from artichoke. An extensive body of research has shown that this substance can play an important role in treating liver disease and help damaged liver tissue to regenerate. The great advantage of using food as medicine is that food is readily available to all of us and can be self-administered with relative safety. Food cures work in a purely holistic way by enhancing the body's natural functions and encouraging it to heal itself.

using this book

The aim of *Food is Medicine* is to provide inspiration and practical advice that will help you to adopt healthy eating habits and to use food in medicinal ways. The book is divided into four parts. The first part – Guide to healing foods – lists more than 140 common foods, their nutrients and their most important medicinal properties. It also identifies seven "star" foods that are renowned for their beneficial properties. Part two – Food for common ailments – specifies the foods that can play a part in treating over 80 common medical conditions. The third part – Healing recipes – is a collection of recipes that use medicinal foods in interesting and delicious combinations. The final part of the book – Diet in practice – offers a practical guide to vitamins and minerals and the foods in which they are found. It also explains how to detoxify your body with a simple diet based on fruit, vegetables, juices and herbal infusions.

Most of the recipes and techniques that I have selected are straightforward to make and use easily available ingredients. The recipes can be used in three different ways:

● As everyday dishes for people who are healthy, but interested in preserving their long-term well-being by incorporating health-giving foods in their diet.

● As remedies for acute and chronic illnesses. The recipes for juices (pages 110–113) and medicinal drinks (pages 117–125) will be the most useful as they are the most medicinally potent.

Food remedies can be used in conjunction with conventional medical treatment to manage or heal a variety of severe or chronic complaints. The time that it takes to witness improvements depends on your ailment and state of health – try to be patient and persevere with food remedies. Illnesses that are stress-related are also amenable to dietary treatment.

● As first-aid treatments and for symptom relief. Some of the foods used in the recipes can alleviate problems such as indigestion and period pain. Others can be applied to the skin as remedies for bites, burns, stings and skin problems, such as eczema, or as beauty treatments.

Some of the medicinal drink recipes contain alcohol in the form of wine or vodka. Although in large quantities alcohol is bad for health, it is an excellent solvent that concentrates the active ingredients of plants. Macerating a herb such as basil in vodka, for example, preserves its medicinal compounds in a form that is easy and convenient to take (basil is good for indigestion, nausea and to ease feelings of bloatedness). Most medicinal drinks that contain alcohol need be taken in only small doses or for a short period of time – just long enough to help a particular symptom or condition. The medicinal infusions and decoctions often fall into the category of traditional herbal medicine rather than dietary remedies. Since all of the medicinal drinks are potent, they should be used with caution and should not be given to children unless the recipe states that this is acceptable. If you are in doubt about whether it is appropriate to treat yourself with herbal or food remedies, or you are worried about a health problem, consult your doctor.

In a few recipes, a little cream may be added to the finished dish – this is entirely optional. If you have a health problem such as lactose intolerance, use soya milk and soya yoghurt instead of milk products. If you suffer from hypertension, high cholesterol, heart disease or diabetes, you should avoid adding sugar, salt and fat to any of the recipes.

selecting and harvesting ingredients

Whenever possible, use organically-grown fruit and vegetables, make sure they are fresh and avoid keeping them in a refrigerator for too long. When buying meat, buy organically-produced, free-range or farm-raised meat; buy small quantities of quality cuts rather than larger amounts of cheaper meat. Try to buy fish on the same day that it is delivered to your fishmonger.

If possible, try to harvest wild ingredients from your garden or local countryside. When picking ingredients, such as borage leaves, nettles and dandelion leaves, choose young plants that are growing away from main roads, rail tracks, and paths that are regularly used by animals. Make sure that you can confidently identify the plants that you need and that what you pick is in good condition and fit for consumption. You can cultivate many herbs, such as camomile, lemon balm, savory, mint, basil, thyme and rosemary, in your garden or in pots on a patio or balcony. When harvesting wild fruit, such as berries, choose bushes and trees that are not exposed to pollution from roads. Collect only undamaged, ripe fruit and don't be tempted to eat it on the spot – it must be washed thoroughly, and preferably cooked.

Pierre Jean Cousin

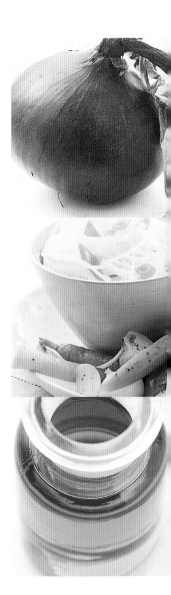
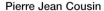

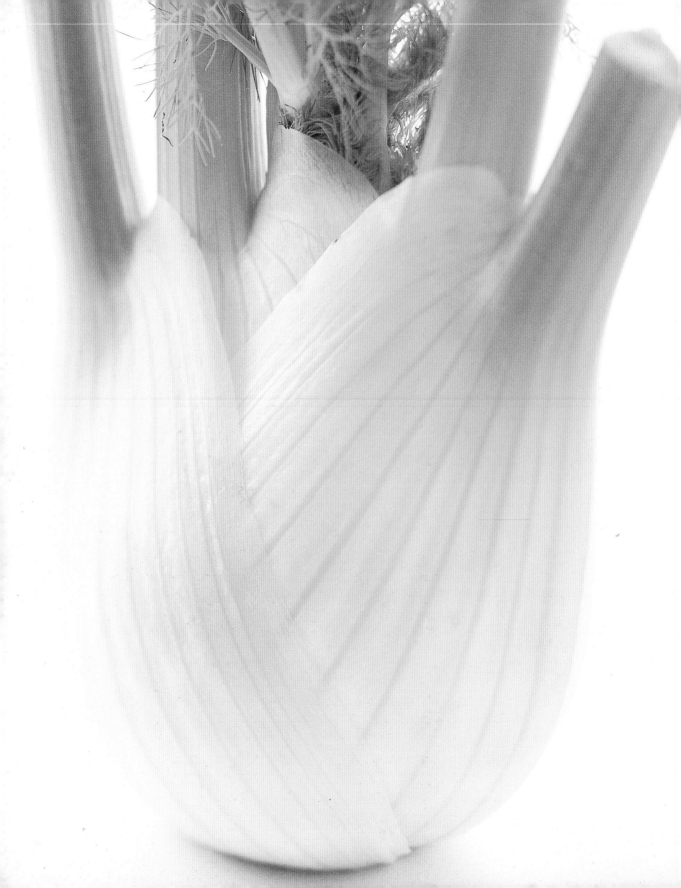

guide to healing foods

Many people consider food as fuel – they need it simply to keep them going through the day. But food can also prevent and treat illness, offering an astounding medicine chest of natural remedies that come with little or no risk. The foods in this section are arranged by type to help you to make informed choices about which specific foods may be beneficial to you. Included are seven star foods – true wonders of nature that we should all include in our diet to boost and protect good health.

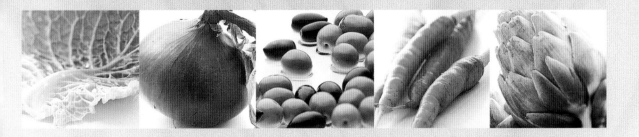

vegetables, cereals and pulses
ROOT VEGETABLES

POTATO

★ VITAMINS B, C, FOLIC ACID, COPPER, PHOSPHORUS, POTASSIUM, SULPHUR, CARBOHYDRATE

● DIGESTIVE SYSTEM Diabetes, gastritis, peptic ulcers,

Potatoes are good for mild digestive problems. Potato juice, mixed with equal amounts of carrot and cabbage juice and a little lemon juice to taste, can ease the symptoms of gastritis and peptic ulcers. The juice or pulp of raw potatoes can be applied directly to burns, insect bites, eczema and boils. Germinated or green potatoes should not be eaten as they may cause stomach upset. *RECIPES chicken breasts with celeriac mash (page 100), dandelion, bacon and potato cakes (page 100), potato and watercress mash (page 103), potatoes with herb sauce (page 105).*

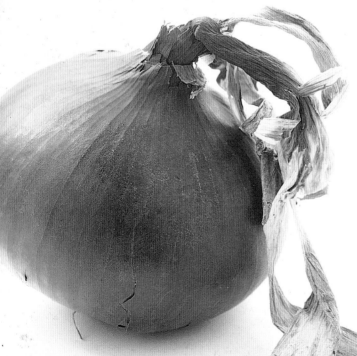

PARSNIP

★ VITAMINS C, FOLIC ACID, E, PHOSPHORUS, POTASSIUM, CARBOHYDRATE, FIBRE

Parsnips belong to the same family as carrots and parsley. They contain small quantities of essential oils (mostly terpenes) that are thought to have anti-cancer properties.

TURNIP

★ VITAMINS A, B, C, FOLIC ACID, CALCIUM, IRON, MAGNESIUM, PHOSPHORUS, POTASSIUM, SULPHUR, NATURAL SUGAR

Turnips, together with several other vegetables, such as broccoli, cabbage, brussels sprouts, cauliflower and swede, are cruciferous (see Broccoli, page 16). Both the root and the young leaves of the turnip can be eaten (the root can be eaten raw, grated in salads). *RECIPES young turnip salad (page 92), pickled turnips (page 114).*

ONION AND SHALLOT

★ VITAMINS A, B, C, MAGNESIUM, PHOSPHORUS, POTASSIUM, SULPHUR COMPOUNDS, BIOFLAVONOIDS, ESSENTIAL OIL, NATURAL SUGAR

● BONES AND JOINTS Arthritis (rheumatoid), gout, rheumatism.

● BLOOD AND CIRCULATION Arteriosclerosis.

● DIGESTIVE SYSTEM Diabetes, diarrhoea.

● IMMUNE SYSTEM Colds, influenza.

● WOMEN'S HEALTH Period pain.

Onions have antibiotic and anti-fungal properties, can block tumour formation, reduce levels of blood cholesterol and prevent blood clots forming. They ease fluid retention and promote the elimination of urea. Onions are beneficial to both the digestive and circulatory systems. They can be juiced or used in a decoction for the treatment of digestive problems, diarrhoea, coughs, colds and flu. Onions can be eaten raw (macerating in olive oil makes them more palatable). Onion juice can be drunk mixed with water or carrot juice; it can also be applied neat to insect stings, warts and boils. *RECIPES onions in cider (page 103).*

BEETROOT

★ VITAMINS A, B, C, IRON, MAGNESIUM, MANGANESE, POTASSIUM, ZINC, ASPARAGIN, BETAINE, BIOFLAVONOIDS, NATURAL SUGAR

● BLOOD AND CIRCULATION Anaemia.

Beetroot is nutritious, easy to digest and a rich source of minerals. It contains betaine, a substance that regulates gastric pH and facilitates digestion. Beetroot can be eaten raw, chopped or grated in salads, or drunk as a juice (one glass per day for a month is the recommended dosage for improving digestive function). The leafy tops of the beetroot plant can be cooked in soups; they are rich in vitamins and minerals and good for the liver.

RECIPES borscht (page 86), beetroot and celery juice (page 113), pickled beetroot (page 114).

CELERIAC

★ VITAMINS A, B, C, IODINE, IRON, MAGNESIUM, MANGANESE, POTASSIUM, ANTIOXIDANTS

● BLOOD AND CIRCULATION Hyperlipidaemia.

Celeriac is the root of a variety of celery plant; it helps to lower levels of blood cholesterol and reduce the risk of bowel cancer.

RECIPES chicken breasts with celeriac mash (page 100).

RADISH (RED AND BLACK)

★ FOLIC ACID, SULPHUR, RAPHANOL, WATER

● BONES AND JOINTS Arthritis (rheumatoid).

● DIGESTIVE SYSTEM Dyspepsia.

● RESPIRATORY SYSTEM Cough, whooping cough.

Although radishes are of poor overall nutritional value, they contain an active ingredient called raphanol that promotes bile flow and the emptying of the gallbladder. There are different types of radish. Black radishes are much larger than the common red variety and contain a greater concentration of raphanol. A combination of carrot and black radish juice is recommended for people with poor liver function and gallbladder problems such as gallstones – mix equal amounts of juice in a 150 ml glass. Both black and red radishes are best eaten raw in salads. A syrup of black radish can be used as an expectorant cough mixture that is appropriate for whooping cough. The young leaves of red radishes contain valuable minerals and are an excellent addition to soups.

RECIPES radish and kumquat salad (page 90), escarole salad (page 93), black radish salad (page 93), black radish syrup (page 124).

LEEK

★ VITAMINS B, C, CALCIUM, IRON, MAGNESIUM, MANGANESE, PHOSPHORUS, POTASSIUM, SILICA, SULPHUR

● BONES AND JOINTS Arthritis (rheumatoid), gout.

● KIDNEYS AND BLADDER Bladder stones.

Leeks belong to the same family as garlic and onion, and contain smaller amounts of the same active ingredients. Leeks are diuretic, laxative, antiseptic and are excellent for a healthy digestive tract. Leek juice can be used externally on abscesses, skin inflammation, stings and bites. A leek macerated in vinegar for 24 hours is an effective remedy for corns and calluses – apply to the affected area overnight and repeat if necessary.

RECIPES buckwheat with leek sauce (page 97), leek and chive mimosa with polenta (page 99), leek syrup (page 124).

continues on page 16

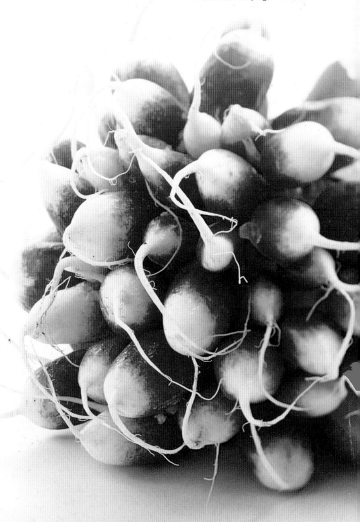

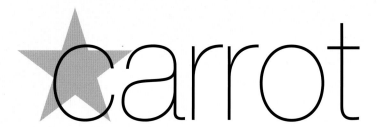

carrot

CARROTS ARE RICH IN ANTIOXIDANTS AND PROTECT THE BODY FROM CERTAIN TYPES OF CANCER. THEY BOOST THE IMMUNE SYSTEM AND ARE USEFUL IN TREATING A RANGE OF AILMENTS, FROM POOR NIGHT VISION TO STOMACH ULCERS.

The properties of carrot

The medicinal properties of carrots were known to the Greeks and Romans. Carrots then were long, thin yellow roots with a strong scent. Modern carrots, which originated in Holland in the 17th century, tend to be orange-coloured, plump and short.

Carrots are one of the most precious vegetables in a medicinal kitchen – they contain vitamin A, folic acid, iron, potassium, magnesium, manganese, sulphur, copper, carotenes and pectin. Their high fibre and fluid content makes them gently laxative and good for constipation, but they also have astringent properties that makes them good for diarrhoea – they can be used as a remedy for either problem in children. A treatment for diarrhoea in adults consists of eating boiled carrots and boiled rice and drinking black tea. The young leaves of carrots are rich in minerals and can be added to soups or cooked with cereals as a tonic for children or people recovering from illness.

Raw carrots inhibit the activity of listeria and salmonella, and thus help to prevent or reduce the risk of food poisoning. Carrots are recommended for chronic fatigue, anaemia, poor immune defences, poor night vision, stomach ulcers and intestinal problems. They can also promote lactation in nursing mothers. Carrot juice contains more medicinally-active ingredients than cooked carrots and the juice is recommended for young children. Raw carrots were traditionally given to horses suffering from bronchitis.

Carrots should be peeled to remove organophosphates (and other artificial residues from pesticides and fertilizers) that may accumulate in the outer part of the vegetable. Where possible, buy organically-grown carrots that are free from organophosphates and fertilizers.

Long-term health benefits

Carrots are an excellent source of antioxidants and are known to have a protective action against lung and other types of cancer. A diet that includes plenty of carrots also lowers unhealthy levels of cholesterol in the blood – preventing the build up of fatty deposits in artery walls – and boosts the body's immune system.

Carrots are a cheap and easily available source of antioxidants and, ideally, they should be consumed two or three times a week either raw in salads (or as snacks) or in juice form.

Medicinal preparations

Carrot seeds can be made into a medicinal infusion (page 118) that stimulates appetite and digestion, and is both diuretic and carminative (relieves flatulence). Externally, carrot juice can be mixed with other ingredients, including cucumber, strawberries and chervil, to make a beauty treatment that rejuvenates the face and neck. An external application of carrot juice can also help to alleviate eczema and acne.

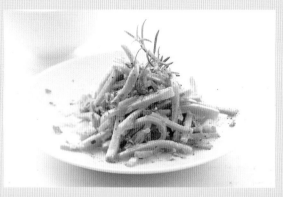

carrots with rosemary

30 g butter
1 red onion, sliced
1 kg carrots, peeled and sliced
1 heaped tablespoon finely chopped rosemary
5 tablespoons fresh cream or yoghurt
Salt and pepper
1 tablespoon chopped parsley

In a saucepan, melt the butter and add the onion, carrots and rosemary. Cover and let the ingredients cook slowly in their own juices for 30 minutes or until the carrots are tender. Add a little water if the saucepan becomes dry. When the carrots are cooked, add the cream or yoghurt and season to taste. Serve sprinkled with parsley.

carrot salad

500 g carrots, grated
Juice of 1 lemon
Juice of 1 orange
Pinch of salt

Mix the ingredients in a large bowl. Cover and chill before serving.

carrot, cabbage and sweet pepper juice

4 medium carrots, roughly chopped
½ cabbage, core removed and quartered
1 red or green pepper, de-seeded
2 small shallots

In a juicer, process the ingredients, adding water if necessary. Chill and serve soon after making.

STAR FOOD PROFILE

- **BLOOD AND CIRCULATION** Anaemia.
- **DIGESTIVE SYSTEM** Diarrhoea, flatulence, peptic ulcers.
- **NERVOUS SYSTEM, MIND AND EMOTIONS** Mental fatigue.
- **SKIN, HAIR AND NAILS** acne, Dermatitis and eczema.

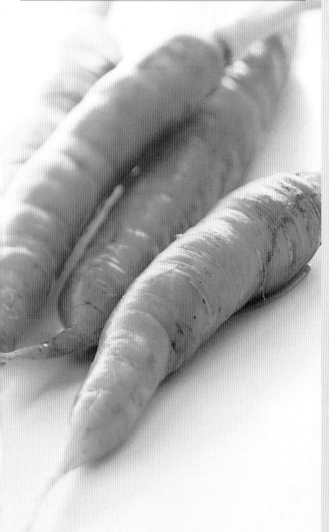

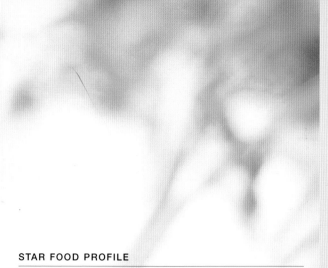

GREEN AND LEAFY VEGETABLES

BROCCOLI

★ VITAMINS A, C, FOLIC ACID, E, CALCIUM, IRON, ZINC

● BLOOD AND CIRCULATION High blood pressure.

Broccoli, together with several other vegetables, such as turnips, cabbage, brussels sprouts, cauliflower and swedes, belong to the cruciferous family. They are rich in antioxidants and are believed to reduce the risk of certain types of cancer, including lung and colon cancer. Avoid overcooking broccoli as approximately half of its beneficial substances may be destroyed in the process.

RECIPES broccoli and green bean juice (page 113).

BRUSSELS SPROUT

★ VITAMIN A, C, FOLIC ACID, E, IRON, POTASSIUM

See Broccoli, above.

RECIPES brussels sprouts with chestnuts (page 104).

CAULIFLOWER

★ VITAMINS C, FOLIC ACID, E, POTASSIUM, ZINC, CAROTENES

● BONES AND JOINTS Arthritis (rheumatoid).

See Broccoli, above.

RECIPES pickled cauliflower (page 114).

GREEN BEAN

★ VITAMIN A, FOLIC ACID, COPPER, PHOSPHORUS, SILICA, CARBOHYDRATE, CHLOROPHYLL

● BONES AND JOINTS Arthritis (rheumatoid), gout, rheumatism.

● KIDNEYS AND BLADDER Kidney stones.

Green beans have diuretic properties which help kidney function and prevent water retention. They stimulate the production of white blood cells (needed to defend the body against infection) and are gently cardio-tonic. For rheumatism, water retention or as a general cardio-tonic, green beans should be eaten every day for a month (the cooking water can be also be drunk or used as a stock for soup). Alternatively, half a glass of green bean juice every morning for four to five weeks has the same medicinal benefits.

RECIPES green bean salad (page 91), green beans with dijon mustard (page 105), green bean and garlic juice (page 113), broccoli and green bean juice (page 113).

CHARD

★ VITAMINS A, B, FOLIC ACID, IRON

Chard is a form of beet that is grown for its green leaves. It has diuretic and laxative properties and is useful for treating kidney and bladder inflammation. The cooked leaves can be used in a poultice for burns, abscesses and boils.

DANDELION

★ VITAMINS A, B, C, FOLIC ACID, CALCIUM, IRON, MANGANESE, POTASSIUM, SILICA, BIOFLAVONOIDS, BITTER PRINCIPLE, CHLOROPHYLL, INULIN

● BLOOD AND CIRCULATION Anaemia, hyperlipidaemia.

● DIGESTIVE SYSTEM Colitis, constipation, gallstones.

● KIDNEYS AND BLADDER Kidney stones.

● SKIN, HAIR AND NAILS Eczema.

Dandelion leaves are recommended for people with poor liver function, gallbladder or kidney stones. The young leaves can be used in salads or cooked in the same way as other green leafy vegetables. When choosing young dandelion plants for salads or soups, include the young flower buds. The fresh sap from the dandelion is said to be an effective topical treatment for verrucae. Dandelion root is widely used in herbal medicine for its diuretic and detoxifying properties.

RECIPES dandelion, bacon and potato cakes (page 100), dandelion infusion (page 117).

NETTLE

★ VITAMINS A, C, CAROTENE, CALCIUM, IRON, MAGNESIUM, POTASSIUM, SILICA, SULPHUR

● BONES AND JOINTS Arthritis (rheumatoid), gout, rheumatism.

● BLOOD AND CIRCULATION Anaemia.

● DIGESTIVE SYSTEM Diarrhoea.

Nettles are a novel addition to many recipes. They are diuretic, astringent and depurative; they promote the elimination of uric acid, stimulate liver function, appetite and bile flow; and they help combat infection. Nettles can be used as a fortifying ingredient in recipes for children and people recovering from illness. They are also good for diminishing menstrual and other types of bleeding. *RECIPES nettle soup (page 88), nettle risotto (page 97), halibut steak and nettle butter (page 101).*

SPINACH

★ VITAMIN C, FOLIC ACID, IRON, ZINC, CAROTENE

Spinach is rich in antioxidants and stimulates pancreas function. The juice is a powerful tonic; an infusion of the seeds is good for mild constipation (cover 10 g of seeds in 250 ml boiling water, infuse for 10 minutes then strain); and the leaves can be used as a topical treatment for burns or eczema. Avoid over-consumption of spinach as it may reduce calcium absorption. People who suffer from gout, arthritis or inflammation of the digestive tract should not eat excessive amounts of spinach.

RECIPES lamb with spinach and lentils (page 99), spicy spinach, prunes and beans (page 101), red mullet with raw spinach salad (page 103).

WATERCRESS

★ VITAMINS A, B, C, E, IODINE, IRON, MANGANESE, PHOSPHORUS, ZINC

● BONES AND JOINTS Arthritis (rheumatoid), rheumatism.

● BLOOD AND CIRCULATION Anaemia.

● DIGESTIVE SYSTEM Intestinal parasites.

● RESPIRATORY SYSTEM Bronchitis.

Watercress stimulates the appetite and has tonic, depurative, diuretic, expectorant and anti-cancer properties. It is good for lack of energy. Watercress leaves or juice can be applied to the skin to ease inflammation, ulcers and boils, eliminate freckles and heal scars. The juice or the cooking water is a good hair tonic.

RECIPES cottage cheese with watercress (page 95), potato and watercress mash (page 103).

SALAD VEGETABLES

LETTUCE

★ VITAMINS A, C, D, FOLIC ACID, E, IRON, MANGANESE, POTASSIUM, ZINC, LACTUCARIUM

● NERVOUS SYSTEM, MIND AND EMOTIONS Insomnia.

During the Middle Ages lettuce was served at the start of a meal in order to stimulate the appetite. Because it is rich in fibre it helps food to pass quickly through the intestines, and aids digestion. Lettuce contains lactucarium, a substance that has sedative and analgesic properties, and is thought to be useful in the treatment of mild insomnia. Lettuce seeds are the most valuable part of the plant from a medicinal perspective. A decoction of the seeds is helpful for asthma, bronchitis, spasmodic cough and insomnia. A decoction of lettuce leaves can be used externally as an anti-inflammatory treatment for conjunctivitis and acne.

RECIPES lettuce and basil juice (page 113), lettuce-seed decoction (page 120).

LAMB'S LETTUCE

★ VITAMINS A, B, C, FOLIC ACID, IRON, CHLOROPHYLL, FIBRE

● BONES AND JOINTS Arthritis (rheumatoid).

● BLOOD AND CIRCULATION Anaemia, arteriosclerosis.

● DIGESTIVE SYSTEM Constipation, gastroenteritis.

● KIDNEYS AND BLADDER Bladder stones.

Lamb's lettuce is recommended for digestive problems. It has detoxifying and slight diuretic properties, it facilitates the elimination of urea (which prevents the formation of uric acid crystals) and is said to be good for respiratory disorders, probably by helping the elimination of mucus. Lamb's lettuce is best eaten raw in salads but can also be cooked or taken in juice form.

ROCKET

★ VITAMINS A, B, C, FOLIC ACID, IRON, CHLOROPHYLL, FIBRE

● DIGESTIVE SYSTEM Dyspepsia.

Rocket was once considered to be an aphrodisiac and its cultivation in monasteries was forbidden. It is widely used in Italian cuisine and can be used in salads or lightly cooked with pasta and ravioli. It has tonic properties and stimulates appetite and digestion.

continues on page 20

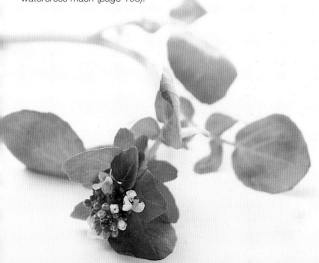

cabbage

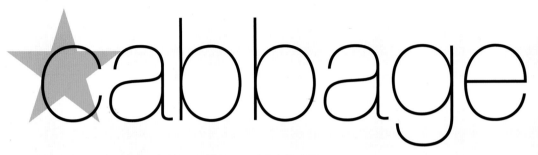

CABBAGE IS A LONG-ESTABLISHED REMEDY FOR A VARIETY OF DIGESTIVE AILMENTS. IT IS ALSO RICH IN ANTIOXIDANTS AND CAN STRENGTHEN THE IMMUNE SYSTEM AND HELP THE BODY TO OVERCOME INFECTION.

The history of cabbage

The therapeutic benefits of the common cabbage have been known and appreciated across Europe for thousands of years: the Slavs, Celts, Basques and Germans all used cabbage for both food and medicine and the Romans considered it to be a panacea for almost any disease. It is thought that cultivation of the cabbage plant may go back as far as the Neolithic period. Cabbage belongs to the cruciferous family of vegetables, which also includes broccoli and turnip. There are many different colours, sizes and varieties of cabbage.

The properties of cabbage

Cabbage is rich in vitamins A, B, C, K and E, potassium, sulphur and copper. It also contains a variety of antioxidants that help to reduce the risk of bowel cancer and cardiovascular disease. Cabbage is anti-inflammatory, diuretic and helps to lower blood sugar. Medicinal uses of cabbage focus on digestive ailments such as gastritis, stomach ulcers, colitis and diverticulitis. Research shows that cabbage juice is an effective treatment for stomach ulcers. A recommended remedy for inflammation of the digestive tract is a small glass of cabbage juice every morning for a few weeks. Cabbage juice is also a natural cleansing and purifying agent.

An immune system stimulant, cabbage is excellent for treating common colds and catarrh, laryngitis and other upper respiratory tract infections. The abundance of sulphur compounds in cabbage also makes it an effective remedy for rheumatism and arthritis. Cabbage contains a small amount of a substance called glucobrassinin which reduces the activity of the thyroid gland. Excessive consumption of cabbage among people who receive insufficient iodine may lead to a mild and rare form of hypothyroidism.

Cabbage in the diet

Many of the active ingredients contained in cabbage are lost in prolonged cooking; raw cabbage and cabbage juice are of greater medicinal value. A good way of eating raw cabbage is chopped and pickled in the form of sauerkraut. This contains a high concentration of lactobacilli – bacteria that are beneficial to the intestines.

Using cabbage externally

Cabbage leaves made into a poultice can be applied externally to heal wounds, fractures, sprains, burns, and joint inflammation caused by rheumatism, arthritis and gout. The juice can be applied to the skin in the treatment of eczema and acne. Cabbage leaves placed on the eyes can relieve local inflammation.

STAR FOOD PROFILE

- **BONES AND JOINTS** Arthritis (rheumatoid), rheumatism.
- **BLOOD AND CIRCULATION** Raynaud's disease.
- **DIGESTIVE SYSTEM** Colitis, diverticulitis, gastritis, peptic ulcers.
- **RESPIRATORY SYSTEM** Asthma, cough.

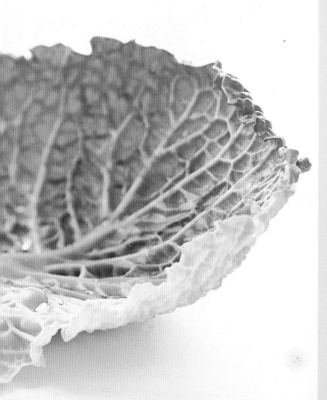

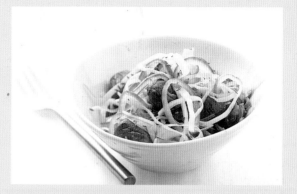

cabbage with chestnuts

This dish goes well with roast pork.

1 medium-sized white cabbage (or red cabbage or Brussels sprouts)
2 tablespoons olive oil
4 medium-sized red onions, sliced
300 g chestnuts, peeled and cooked
To serve: cumin seeds

Chop the cabbage into thin strips, then blanch in salted, boiling water for a few minutes. In another large pan, soften the onions in the olive oil over a low heat, then add the cabbage and chestnuts, and cook for a further 5 minutes. Sprinkle over some cumin seeds before serving hot.

cabbage, carrot and blueberry juice

2 parts fresh cabbage juice
2 parts fresh carrot juice
1 part blueberry juice

Combine the juices thoroughly. Chill and serve.

CELERY

★ VITAMINS A, B, C, CALCIUM, MAGNESIUM, MANGANESE, POTASSIUM, ESSENTIAL OIL

● BONES AND JOINTS gout, Rheumatism.

● KIDNEYS AND BLADDER Kidney or bladder stones.

● IMMUNE SYSTEM Sore throat.

Celery is beneficial for digestive problems and poor appetite. It is best eaten raw in salads or juiced with carrots or green vegetables and is particularly easy to digest in soup form. Fresh celery juice is antiseptic so it can help to ease mouth ulcers and sore throats. The juice can also be mixed with an equal amount of carrot juice and applied to the skin to promote healing. Celery is very low in calories so it is a useful part of a weight-loss diet.

RECIPES celery with wine and herbs (page 104), cabbage, carrot and celery juice (page 113), beetroot and celery juice (page 113).

CUCUMBER

★ VITAMINS A, B, C, IODINE, MANGANESE, SULPHUR

● BONES AND JOINTS Gout, rheumatism.

● DIGESTIVE SYSTEM Ulcerative colitis.

Cucumbers have a very high water content; they are diuretic, anti-inflammatory, help to dissolve uric acid and are good for intestinal health. They should be eaten with the skin on (whenever possible buy organically produced, unwaxed cucumbers). Cucumber flesh or juice can be used externally to reduce inflammation and to hydrate and protect the skin. A face mask can be made from blending 1 tablespoon of fresh cream with equal amounts of cucumber, melon and pumpkin seeds in a food processor. The cream should be applied to the face, left for 30 minutes and then rinsed off.

RECIPES pineapple and cucumber salad (page 93), cucumber salad (page 93), rice with cucumber balls (page 103), cucumber and lettuce heart juice (page 113).

PEPPER

★ VITAMINS A, C, ANTIOXIDANTS

● BONES AND JOINTS Rheumatism.

● DIGESTIVE SYSTEM Diarrhoea, dyspepsia, wind.

The colour of a pepper – green, yellow or red – indicates its stage of maturity. Sweet peppers can be eaten raw in salads and grilled or roasted in a variety of Mediterranean dishes. Hot peppers are used in spicy dishes such as curry; they contain up to 1 per cent capsaicin, a pungent-smelling and -tasting substance that is beneficial for the heart and circulation.

RECIPES stuffed peppers (page 98).

TOMATO

★ VITAMINS A, B, C, FOLIC ACID, TRACE ELEMENTS, ANTIOXIDANTS,

● BONES AND JOINTS Arthritis (rheumatoid), rheumatism.

● DIGESTIVE SYSTEM Cholecystitis, constipation, gallstones.

● KIDNEYS AND BLADDER Bladder stones.

Tomatoes help to dissolve urea, preventing the formation of uric acid crystals. They reduce inflammation of the digestive tract and bacterial activity in the bowel. Many commercially available tomatoes are grown too quickly in hot-houses or are genetically modified. Organically-produced varieties of tomato offer greater medicinal benefits.

RECIPES tomato coulis (page 97), polenta with basil tomato sauce (page 99), celery and tomato juice (page 112).

COURGETTE

★ VITAMINS A, B, C, MAGNESIUM, PHOSPHORUS, POTASSIUM, ZINC, CAROTENES

● DIGESTIVE SYSTEM Dyspepsia, gastroenteritis.

● NERVOUS SYSTEM, MIND AND EMOTIONS Insomnia.

Courgettes are gentle on the intestines, mildly laxative, diuretic and can alleviate bladder and kidney inflammation. They are recommended for diabetic people who manage their illness through diet. Courgettes can be eaten raw in salads or lightly cooked. Courgette juice can be mixed with other vegetable juices and drunk daily. The juice (or the mashed flesh) can be applied to the skin as a remedy for inflammation and abscesses – add clay to make a beauty mask.

RECIPES courgette cake (page 97).

SALAD LEAVES

★ VITAMINS B, C, FOLIC ACID, K, IRON, MAGNESIUM, BIOFLAVONOIDS

Salad leaves, such as chicory, escarole, frisée and endive, have mild diuretic properties and contain a bitter compound that is good for the liver and gallbladder. They are an important source of nutrients. Chicory root may be dried and roasted and used as a caffeine-free alternative to coffee. Endive is grown without light and has little nutritional value.

RECIPES escarole salad (page 93).

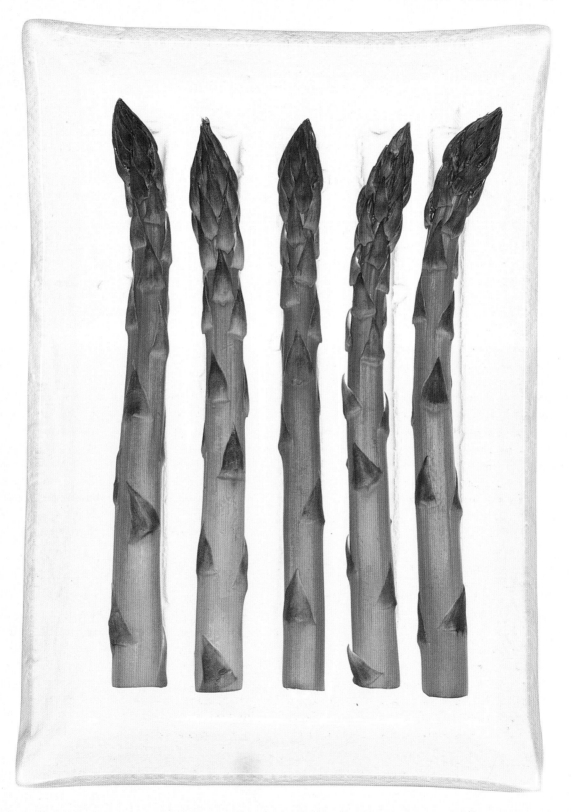

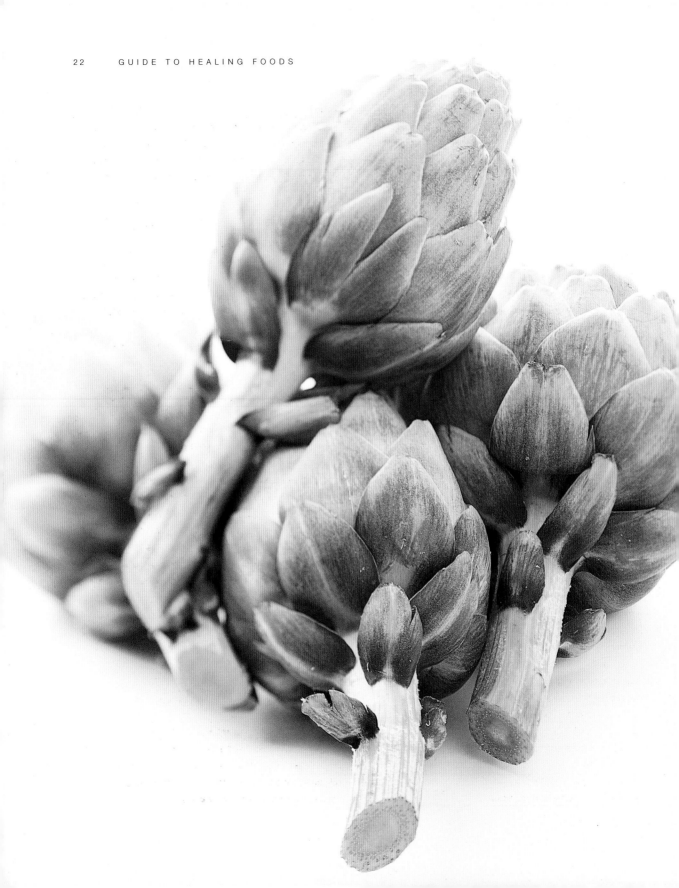

GOURMET VEGETABLES

ASPARAGUS

★ VITAMINS A, B, C, FOLIC ACID, COPPER, FLUORIDE, MANGANESE, POTASSIUM, ASPARAGINE

● BLOOD AND CIRCULATION Arteriosclerosis, high blood pressure, hyperlipidaemia.

● DIGESTIVE SYSTEM Constipation.

Asparagus is diuretic, low in calories, and, owing to its high fibre content, is good for intestinal health. It inhibits bacterial activity in the intestines, promotes lactation and has anti-cancer properties. Asparagine is an active ingredient in asparagus that has an irritant effect – for this reason, asparagus should be avoided by people suffering from ailments that involve inflammation, such as gout, rheumatism and cystitis. Asparagus may be grated and eaten raw in salads, although it is more commonly boiled or steamed until tender.

RECIPES warm asparagus salad (page 93), asparagus syrup (page 125).

ARTICHOKE

★ VITAMINS A, B, C, IRON, MANGANESE, PHOSPHORUS, CYNARIN

Artichoke contains substances that are proven to be beneficial to the kidneys (by promoting diuresis) and to the liver (by promoting detoxification). Artichoke improves the secretion of bile and its emulsification and therefore aids the digestion of fat. It also helps to lower levels of blood cholesterol. Some types of young artichokes can be eaten raw in salad; other varieties should be steamed or boiled (the cooking water contains most of the bitter active ingredient and should be drunk for maximum benefit). An infusion made with artichoke leaves can alleviate liver and kidney problems. Artichoke buds are detoxifying and can help to alleviate rheumatism, gout and water retention. Nursing mothers should avoid artichoke – it makes breast milk taste bitter and slows down the production of milk.

RECIPES Roman-style artichoke (page 95), artichoke-leaf wine (page 122), artichoke-leaf tincture (page 124).

JERUSALEM ARTICHOKE

★ VITAMINS A, C, TRACE ELEMENTS, INULIN

● DIGESTIVE SYSTEM Constipation, dyspepsia, gastritis.

Jerusalem artichoke is a nutritious vegetable that is often over-looked in cooking – it is recommended for people with diabetes. To retain its nutritional value, grate the Jerusalem artichoke in salads, steam or boil lightly; keep the cooking water for use in soups.

AVOCADO

★ VITAMINS A, B, C, FOLIC ACID, ESSENTIAL AMINO ACIDS

Avocado, a fruit that is widely used as a vegetable, inhibits certain types of bacteria in the intestine and helps to regulate cholesterol (studies suggest that it may lower blood cholesterol levels). Mashed avocado flesh can be applied to the skin as a treatment for aging or dryness, or made into a beauty mask by combining with egg white, egg yolk or honey.

RECIPES avocado dressing (page 89), avocado tartar (page 95).

FENNEL

★ VITAMINS A, B COMPLEX, PHOSPHORUS, POTASSIUM, SULPHUR, ESSENTIAL OILS

● DIGESTIVE SYSTEM Abdominal cramp and colic, nausea.

● NERVOUS SYSTEM, MIND AND EMOTIONS Headache.

● WOMEN'S HEALTH Period pain.

Fennel stimulates appetite, facilitates digestion and promotes the secretion of bile. It is best eaten raw in salads (it goes very well with radicchio) but is also excellent cooked. If fennel is eaten in combination with pulses, it facilitates their digestion and prevents the formation of digestive gases. An infusion of fennel seeds has the same medicinal effects as eating the bulb. Fennel can be eaten by breastfeeding mothers to stimulate the baby's appetite and to prevent colic and digestive problems.

RECIPES fennel and radicchio salad (page 91), fennel with wine (page 104), fennel infusion (page 117), corn-hair and fennel-seed decoction (page 119), fennel-seed decoction (page 120).

SEAWEED

★ VITAMIN C, CALCIUM, IRON, MAGNESIUM, PHOSPHORUS, POTASSIUM, SODIUM

● BLOOD AND CIRCULATION Atherosclerosis, high blood pressure.

Seaweed has bactericidal and anti-cancer properties, it boosts the immune system, heals ulcers, reduces levels of cholesterol in the blood, lowers blood pressure, thins the blood and helps to prevent stroke and other cardiovascular diseases.

SALSIFY

★ CARBOHYDRATE, INULIN

● **BONES AND JOINTS** Arthritis (rheumatoid), gout.

● **DIGESTIVE SYSTEM** Diabetes.

● **SKIN, HAIR AND NAILS** Eczema.

Salsify belongs to the daisy family and has a long root similar to that of a parsnip. Salsify is often overlooked in cooking. It has detoxifying properties and is good for liver and kidney function. When peeling salsify, plunge it in cold water with the juice of half a lemon (or 2 tablespoons of vinegar) to prevent it turning black. The juice is a natural remedy for verrucae – apply it directly to the skin.

RECIPES salsify (page 104).

PUMPKIN

★ FOLIC ACID, ANTIOXIDANTS, CAROTENE

● **DIGESTIVE SYSTEM** Diabetes, dysentery, dyspepsia.

● **KIDNEYS AND BLADDER** Cystitis.

● **NERVOUS SYSTEM, MIND AND EMOTIONS** Insomnia.

Pumpkins are low in calories, high in water, calming and cooling. The juice is a good laxative, and the flesh can be applied to the skin to calm inflammation, burns and abscesses. Pumpkin seeds, peeled and cooked in water or milk, can ease insomnia and cystitis. The roasted seeds are a good source of essential fatty acids, magnesium, phosphorus, zinc and potassium.

RECIPES baked pumpkin strudel (page 101), pumpkin in syrup (page 106).

AUBERGINE

★ VITAMINS A, B, C, CALCIUM, COPPER, MAGNESIUM, MANGANESE, PHOSPHORUS, POTASSIUM, ZINC, BIOFLAVONOIDS

● **DIGESTIVE SYSTEM** Constipation.

Aubergine is a low-calorie vegetable that is widely used in Mediterranean, Indian and oriental cuisine. It has laxative properties, it calms the mind and gently stimulates liver and pancreas function. The unripe aubergine is slightly toxic. Aubergine should always be cooked before eating – sprinkling salt on slices of aubergine 1 hour before cooking can reduce the water content and the amount of fat that is absorbed during cooking. Aubergine leaves are cooling and anti-inflammatory, they can be applied to burns, abscesses and eczema.

RECIPES pepper and aubergine salad (page 89), grilled salmon with aubergine sauce (page 97).

MUSHROOM

★ COPPER, IODINE, MANGANESE, POTASSIUM, SELENIUM, ZINC, PROTEIN

Mushrooms have stimulant properties and can help to strengthen the immune system. They are a useful source of protein in a meat-free diet. Mushrooms harvested from the wild should be identified as edible and cooked thoroughly before eating (they should not be added raw to salads). Some varieties are highly toxic.

RECIPES buckwheat pancakes with field mushrooms (page 98).

PULSES

BEAN (RED KIDNEY, HARICOT, FLAGEOLET, BORLOTTI)

★ CALCIUM, IRON, MAGNESIUM, PHOSPHORUS, POTASSIUM, CARBOHYDRATE, FIBRE, PROTEIN

● **DIGESTIVE SYSTEM** Diabetes.

Beans are good for people with diabetes or weak liver function, but should be eaten in moderation by gout and rheumatism sufferers. Germinated beans are particularly tasty and nutritious. Beans are easier to digest if they are cooked and eaten with aromatic herbs such as garlic, thyme and bay leaves. Red kidney beans contain a substance that can upset the stomach – boiling them vigorously for 15 minutes renders this substance harmless.

RECIPES mediterranean bean salad (page 90), spicy spinach, prunes and beans (page 101), beans with carrots and onions (page 104).

BROAD BEAN

★ CALCIUM, IRON, MAGNESIUM, PHOSPHORUS, POTASSIUM, CARBOHYDRATE, PROTEIN

● **DIGESTIVE SYSTEM** Diarrhoea, dysentery.

Broad beans are good for the kidneys and bladder. An infusion of broad bean flowers (steep a handful of flowers in 150 ml of boiling water for 10 minutes) eases pain from kidney stones and sciatica.

RECIPES broad bean soup (page 86).

LENTIL

★ FOLIC ACID, CALCIUM, IRON, POTASSIUM, PROTEIN, CARBOHYDRATE

● **BLOOD AND CIRCULATION** Atherosclerosis, high blood pressure.

● **DIGESTIVE SYSTEM** Diabetes, constipation.

Lentils are nutritious, digestible, regulate colon function and should be eaten frequently as part of a healthy diet. They are recommended for pregnant women and people on a cholesterol-lowering diet.

Lentils and other pulses may help to inhibit cancerous growth. *RECIPES red lentil soup (page 89), lamb with spinach and lentils (page 99).*

PEA

★ VITAMIN C, FOLIC ACID, IRON, PHOSPHORUS, CARBOHYDRATE, FIBRE, PROTEIN

Peas are an energy-providing food that has tonic properties and helps to regulate bowel function.

RECIPES peas with bacon pieces (page 104).

CHICKPEA

★ CALCIUM, IRON, MAGNESIUM, PHOSPHORUS, POTASSIUM, SILICA, CARBOHYDRATE, PROTEIN

● DIGESTIVE SYSTEM Intestinal parasites.

Chickpeas are a staple food in many Mediterranean and North African countries. They are nutritious, easy to digest and have antiseptic and diuretic properties. They are good for inflammation of the urinary tract and for poor digestion.

RECIPES chickpea broth (page 86).

SOYA

★ VITAMINS A, B COMPLEX, FOLIC ACID, CALCIUM, MAGNESIUM, CARBOHYDRATE, FIBRE, LECITHIN, PROTEIN

Soya in the form of miso, tofu, beans and bean sprouts is a staple food in the East. Most soya is now genetically modified. Soya bean sprouts are anti-inflammatory, can reduce stomach acidity and relieve rheumatism.

CEREALS

BUCKWHEAT

★ VITAMIN A, PROTEIN, SELENIUM, CARBO- HYDRATE, IMPORTANT AMINO ACIDS AND RUTIN

Buckwheat contains rutin – a substance that protects the heart – and is free of gluten, a protein that is insoluble in water and can be difficult to eliminate. It is a useful alternative to wheat for people who suffer from celiac disease or are gluten-intolerant. Buckwheat flour can be used instead of wheat

flour during illnesses characterized by mucus production (gluten has a glue-like quality and acts in a similar way to mucus).

RECIPES buckwheat with leek sauce (page 97), buckwheat pancakes with field mushrooms (page 98).

CORN

★ VITAMINS A, B, E, IRON, MAGNESIUM, PHOSPHORUS, POTASSIUM, CARBOHYDRATE, FIBRE, POLYUNSATURATED FAT, SOME FATTY ACIDS

Corn should be eaten from the cob or as coarse-ground polenta. Other forms of corn are depleted of nutrients by milling and processing. Corn is suitable for people with gluten intolerance. It is said to be a gentle moderator of the thyroid gland. Cold-pressed corn oil is rich in polyunsaturated fat (mostly oleic acid) and helps to reduce high cholesterol levels. It is good in salad dressings but is rapidly damaged by heat and loses its therapeutic value when used in cooking and frying. Organic corn oil is difficult to find.

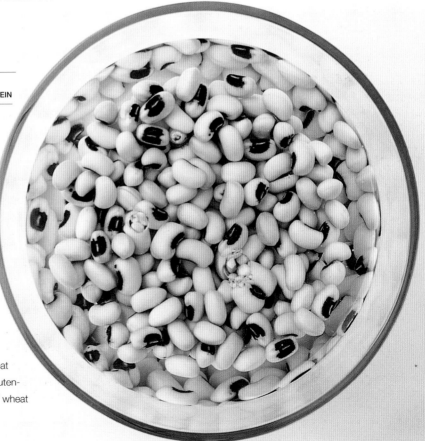

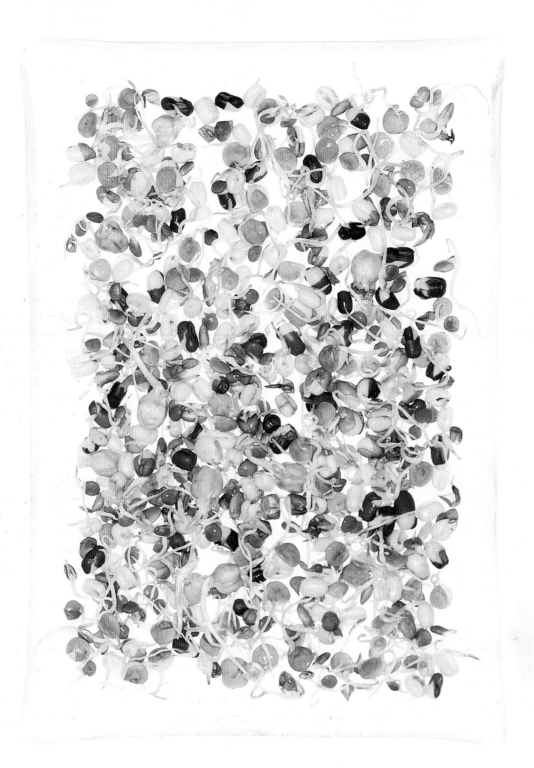

RECIPES polenta with basil tomato sauce (page 99), corn-hair and fennel-seed decoction (page 119)

MILLET

★ IRON, MAGNESIUM, PHOSPHORUS, SILICA, CARBOHYDRATE, FIBRE, PROTEIN

Millet is a useful cereal for people who need to follow a gluten-free diet. It also eases fatigue, has a balancing effect upon the nervous system and is recommended during pregnancy and recovery from illness. Millet increases in volume when cooked in water – because it is very filling, is a useful part of a weight-reducing diet.

RECIPES chicken, millet, barley and celeriac pilaff (page 101).

BARLEY

★ VITAMINS B, E, CALCIUM, COPPER, IODINE, IRON, MAGNESIUM, POTASSIUM, CARBOHYDRATE, FIBRE, L-TRYPTOPHAN

● DIGESTIVE SYSTEM Diarrhoea, dyspepsia.

● NERVOUS SYSTEM, MIND AND EMOTIONS Mild insomnia.

● WOMEN'S HEALTH Premenstrual syndrome.

Barley is good for the digestive and nervous systems, and contains L-tryptophan, an amino acid that is useful in the treatment of mild insomnia and premenstrual syndrome. It also lowers blood sugar and contains hordenine, a substance with cardio-tonic and anti-diarrhoeic properties. A variety of enzymes that can relieve dyspepsia and hyperacidity can be found in germinated barley. As cooking destroys these enzymes, the best way to benefit from the medicinal properties of this cereal is to drink barley water made from germinated barley (page 121). The whole barley grain – germinated if possible – should be eaten for maximum nutritional and health benefits (the polished grain is of little therapeutic value).

RECIPES barley and fruit porridge (page 69), chickpea broth (page 86), chicken, millet, barley and celeriac pilaff (page 101), barley infusion (page 118), barley water (page 121).

OAT

★ FOLIC ACID, CALCIUM, IRON, MAGNESIUM, PHOSPHORUS, POTASSIUM, SODIUM, CARBOHYDRATE, FATTY ACIDS, FIBRE, PROTEIN

● DIGESTIVE SYSTEM Diabetes.

● NERVOUS SYSTEM, MIND AND EMOTIONS Depression, insomnia, mental fatigue.

Oats are nutritious and help to lower levels of cholesterol in the body. They have diuretic properties, stimulate thyroid function and are helpful for people who have diabetes. A tincture of oats (*Avena sativa*) is often prescribed by herbalists and homeopaths for insomnia, mild depression and mental fatigue.

RECIPES barley and fruit porridge (page 69).

RICE

★ VITAMINS A, B COMPLEX, MINERALS AND TRACE ELEMENTS, CARBOHYDRATE, FIBRE, PROTEIN

● DIGESTIVE SYSTEM Diarrhoea, diabetes, diverticulitis.

Rice is an energy-providing food that helps lower blood pressure and has astringent properties. The water in which rice is cooked (rice water) is a remedy for mild diarrhoea: in Vietnam, a cup of rice is soaked in a mixture of water and honey, strained and stir-fried in a wok without oil; then, when the rice has coloured, 2 litres of water are added and the rice is simmered until overcooked. The resulting water is drunk as a diarrhoea remedy. The same recipe can be used as an energy-providing drink for convalescents. Rice is suitable for people on a gluten-free diet. Because polished white rice has lost most of its important ingredients it is preferable to eat organically-produced brown rice. Macrobiotic diets based on brown rice are not recommended for children or menopausal women as they may lead to calcium and iron deficiency.

RECIPES nettle risotto (page 97), stuffed peppers (page 98), rice with cucumber balls (page 103).

WHEAT

★ VITAMINS A, B, E, CARBOHYDRATE, FIBRE, PROTEIN

Wheat is the staple food of the West. Unfortunately, extensive processing and genetic modification have meant that wheat is largely stripped of its nutritious and healing potential. Wheat that is allowed to germinate has increased vitamin and protein content. Wheat bran contains enzymes that facilitate digestion and ease dyspepsia and hyperacidity.

RECIPES taboule (page 94).

RYE

★ CALCIUM, IRON, POTASSIUM, SULPHUR, CARBOHYDRATE, FIBRE

● BLOOD AND CIRCULATION Arteriosclerosis, high blood pressure.

Rye contains a substance that reduces blood viscosity and helps to maintain healthy heart function. The rate of cardiovascular problems has been found to be low in populations where rye is eaten as a staple food.

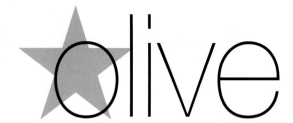

olive

OLIVES FORM A MAJOR PART OF THE MEDITERRANEAN DIET AND, IN CONJUNCTION WITH A LOW INTAKE OF ANIMAL FAT, ARE THOUGHT TO BE IMPORTANT IN REGULATING BLOOD CHOLESTEROL LEVELS AND REDUCING THE RISK OF CARDIOVASCULAR DISEASE.

The properties of olives

There are numerous references to olive trees in the Bible and it is thought that olives were cultivated in Syria around 6000 years ago. Today, major olive producers include Italy, Greece, France, Spain, Portugal, Turkey, Israel, Australia, Africa and many Middle Eastern countries.

Olives contain vitamins A and E, phosphorus, potassium, magnesium, manganese, antioxidants, oleic and linoleic acid. Black olives are easier to digest and have a higher vitamin and antioxidant content than green olives. Only the black olive is edible in its natural state; green olives are washed repeatedly in brine to remove their bitter taste.

Research has demonstrated that people who follow a Mediterranean diet – which is rich in olives and olive oil, and low in animal fat – have a low incidence of cardiovascular disease compared to people who eat a high proportion of animal fat. Studies show that the high oleic acid content in olive oil helps to regulate the balance between high-density lipoprotein (the "good" type of cholesterol) and low-density lipoprotein (the "bad" type of cholesterol) in the blood. This prevents fatty deposits being laid down in the arteries and reduces the risk of atherosclerosis and other types of cardiovascular disease.

Olives are also good for treating diabetes, constipation and gallstones. A remedy for constipation and gallstones is 2 tablespoons of cold-pressed olive oil taken every morning on an empty stomach (an equal amount of lemon juice can be added). The leaves of the olive tree can be used as a remedy for high blood pressure, atherosclerosis, bladder stones, diabetes and angina: bring 50 g dried leaves (or 80 g fresh leaves) and 1 litre of water to the boil. Cover and allow to infuse for 10 minutes and then strain. Drink 150 ml of this decoction three or four times a day. Olive oil has been used as a skin treatment for centuries; it is thought to be invaluable in relieving psoriasis, dry skin and eczema.

Choosing olive oil

Olive oil is traditionally obtained by crushing olives in a stone mill. However, modern extraction techniques have superseded traditional ones and centrifugal or chemical methods are now the most widely used.

The best olive oil to buy is first cold-pressed extra virgin oil. Although the taste and colour may vary from one country to another, or from year to year, this oil is the most nutritious. Try to avoid buying semi-fine or refined olive oil. Check that olive oil falls into one of the following categories:

● Extra virgin olive oil: this is obtained from the first cold pressing of the olives; it is low in acidity (below 1 per cent) and is perfect for medicinal purposes and use in salads.
● Fine virgin olive oil: this is obtained from the second pressing of the olives. Although it has a higher acidity, the taste and medicinal qualities are good.

STAR FOOD PROFILE

- **BLOOD AND CIRCULATION** Angina, atherosclerosis, high blood pressure.
- **DIGESTIVE SYSTEM** Constipation, diabetes, gallstones.
- **KIDNEYS AND BLADDER** Bladder stones.
- **SKIN, HAIR AND NAILS** Dermatitis and eczema.

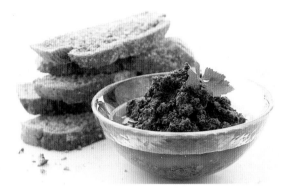

black olive tapenade

200 g black olives, stoned
2–3 cloves garlic, peeled
150 g capers
100 g anchovy fillet, soaked in milk for 10 minutes
1 teaspoon Dijon mustard
2 tablespoons olive oil

Blend the ingredients to a thick paste in a food processor. Serve on toast or with salads or pasta.

aromatic olive oil

Use in vinaigrette and marinades or to brush food prior to cooking.

6 sprigs thyme
1–2 sprigs rosemary
1 sprig sweet marjoram
1 teaspoon black peppercorns
3 cloves garlic, peeled and left whole
2 shallots, left whole
6 bay leaves
1 litre olive oil

Sterilize a pickling jar (page 114), then place all the ingredients into the jar and seal. Leave for 1 month.

green olives and lemon

400 g green olives in brine
Lemon preserved in salt (page 39)
Several small thyme sprigs
Cold-pressed olive oil (see recipe method for amount)
50 ml dry white wine

Drain the olives, setting aside half the brine. In a pickling jar, arrange the olives and lemons in alternate layers. Add the thyme sprigs. Mix the brine with an equal amount of olive oil and the wine. Pour this over the olives and lemons so that they are covered. Tightly seal the jar and leave for 2 or 3 weeks before using as a starter or with salad.

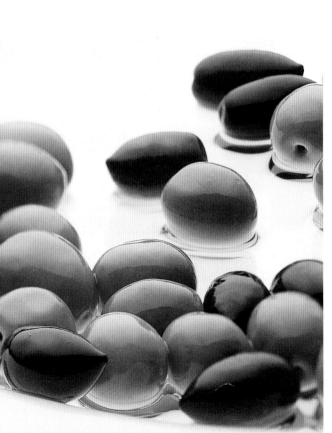

fruits and nuts

EXOTIC FRUIT

COCONUT

★ NATURAL SUGAR, PALMITIC AND OLEIC ACIDS, PROTEIN

Coconut is an excellent protein-based, between-meal snack. It has slight diuretic and laxative properties. The milk can be used to treat stomach ulcers and gastritis.

DATE

★ VITAMINS A, B, D, CALCIUM, MAGNESIUM, POTASSIUM, NATURAL SUGAR

● BLOOD AND CIRCULATION Anaemia,

● RESPIRATORY SYSTEM Bronchitis,

● NERVOUS SYSTEM, MIND AND EMOTIONS Mental fatigue,

Dates may help to prevent cancer. They are a traditional remedy for tuberculosis. In North Africa, respiratory problems are treated with powdered or boiled date stones.
RECIPE banana and date salad (page 106).

FIG

★ VITAMINS A, B, C, FOLIC ACID, CALCIUM, COPPER, IRON, MANGANESE, POTASSIUM, ZINC, NATURAL SUGAR

● DIGESTIVE SYSTEM Constipation, dyspepsia, gastritis, gingivitis.

● RESPIRATORY SYSTEM Bronchitis.

● IMMUNE SYSTEM Sore throat.

Figs are laxative and slightly diuretic. For constipation, cook 4–5 fresh figs in milk with 2 dates and a few raisins – eat for breakfast. For respiratory problems, boil 120 g fresh figs in 1 litre water for 15 minutes, strain and drink. This mixture can also be used as a gargle for sore throats or gingivitis. Figs are good for pregnant women, people recovering from illness and the elderly.
RECIPES fresh figs with raspberry cheese (page 109)

BANANA

★ VITAMINS A, B, FOLIC ACID, E, IODINE, IRON, MAGNESIUM, POTASSIUM, ZINC, CARBOHYDRATE, TRYPTOPHAN

Bananas have antacid and mild antibacterial properties. Consult your doctor about eating bananas if you suffer from diabetes.
RECIPE banana and date salad (page 106).

GUAVA

★ VITAMIN C, POTASSIUM, SULPHUR, CAROTENE, NATURAL SUGAR

● DIGESTIVE SYSTEM Dyspepsia.

Guava has astringent properties and is good for digestion. However, the unripe fruit is difficult to digest and the seeds should not be eaten by people with intestinal problems.

KUMQUAT

★ VITAMIN C, CITRUS FLAVONOIDS, NATURAL SUGAR

Kumquats have the same properties as oranges (page 33).
RECIPES radish and kumquat salad (page 90).

LYCHEE

★ VITAMINS B, C, MAGNESIUM, PHOSPHORUS, POTASSIUM, BIOFLAVONOIDS, NATURAL SUGAR

Lychees stimulate digestion and are slightly astringent. For abdominal pain, drink a decoction of lychee seeds.
RECIPES lychee fruit salad (page 106), lychee-seed decoction (page 120).

MANGO

★ VITAMINS A, B, C, PHOSPHORUS, SULPHUR, CAROTENES, NATURAL SUGAR

● DIGESTIVE SYSTEM Colitis, diarrhoea, ulcerative colitis.

Mango has an astringent effect on the gut which means that it promotes contractions and enhances digestive processes.

PINEAPPLE

★ VITAMINS A, B, C, CITRIC, FOLIC AND MALIC ACIDS, MAGNESIUM, POTASSIUM, BROMELAIN, NATURAL SUGAR

● BONES AND JOINTS Arthritis (rheumatism), gout.

● BLOOD AND CIRCULATION Arteriosclerosis.

● DIGESTIVE SYSTEM Dyspepsia.

Pineapple contains bromelain enzymes that reduce inflammation,

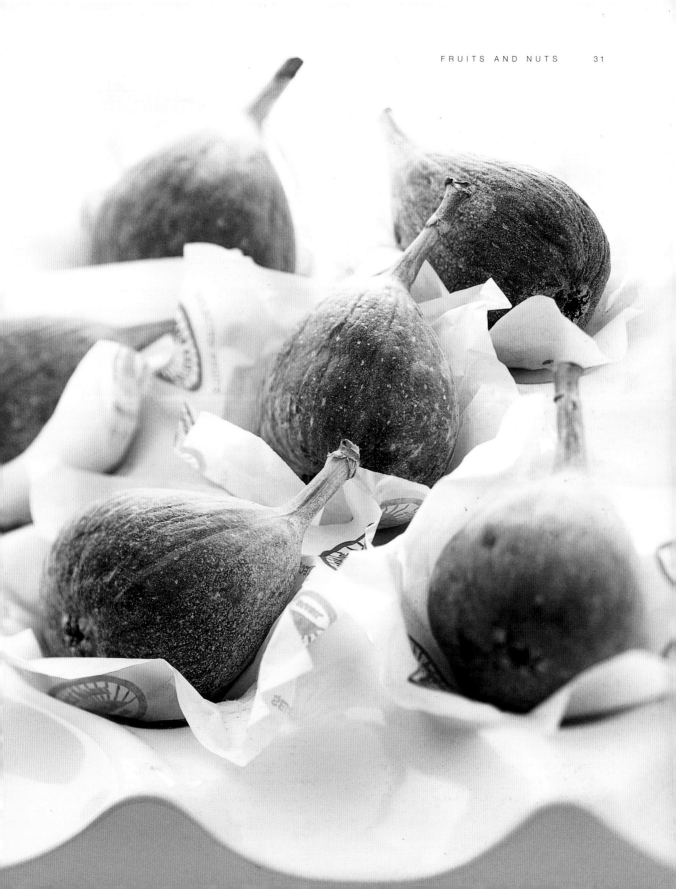

aid digestion and help to break down proteins. Bromelain is used to make various medicines, including anti-inflammatory drugs; it is most concentrated in the core of the pineapple.

RECIPES *pineapple and cucumber salad (page 93).*

PAPAYA

★ VITAMINS A, B, C, POTASSIUM, NATURAL SUGAR, PAPAIN

Papaya contains papain, an enzyme that aids the digestive process by facilitating the breakdown of protein. Papaya is useful for reducing fever.

RECIPES *baked papaya with ginger (page 109).*

SOFT FRUIT AND BERRIES

APRICOT

★ VITAMINS A, B, C, IRON, MAGNESIUM, MANGANESE, PHOSPHORUS, POTASSIUM, NATURAL SUGAR

● BLOOD AND CIRCULATION Anaemia.

● NERVOUS SYSTEM, MIND AND EMOTIONS Mental fatigue, mild anxiety, insomnia.

Apricots have a balancing effect on the nervous system. Both fresh and dried apricots are beneficial for pregnant women, people recovering from illness and elderly people.

RECIPES *poached apricots with cardamom (page 109), apricot, lime and mint juice (page 111).*

GRAPE AND RAISIN

★ VITAMINS A, B, C, CALCIUM, IODINE, MANGANESE, POTASSIUM, SODIUM, BIOFLAVONOIDS, NATURAL SUGAR

● BONES AND JOINTS Arthritis (rheumatoid), gout.

● SKIN, HAIR AND NAILS Dermatitis and eczema.

Grapes are diuretic, detoxifying and laxative. They promote the elimination of uric acid and enhance liver function and bile flow. Black grapes are rich in bioflavonoids, particularly quercetin, which is good for the heart and circulation. Raisins are recommended as a snack for children, pregnant women, convalescents and elderly people. A cold-pressing of grape pips (grape seed oil) is rich in polyunsaturated fatty acids and good for cardiovascular health.

RECIPES *autumn fruit compote (page 108).*

GOOSEBERRY

★ VITAMINS A, B, C, IRON, PHOSPHORUS, POTASSIUM, MALIC AND CITRIC ACIDS, NATURAL SUGAR

● BONES AND JOINTS Arthritis (rheumatoid), gout.

Gooseberries are laxative and diuretic. They stimulate liver function and ease inflammation of the digestive and urinary tracts.

PEACH

★ VITAMINS A, B, C, COPPER, MAGNESIUM, PHOSPHORUS, POTASSIUM, ZINC, NATURAL SUGAR

● DIGESTIVE SYSTEM Dyspepsia.

● KIDNEYS AND BLADDER Bladder stones.

Peaches are diuretic and laxative. Peach blossom is traditionally used to make an infusion or syrup that has calming and laxative properties (suitable for children). An infusion of peach leaves has an even stronger purgative effect. Fresh peach juice may be applied to the skin as a beauty treatment.

RECIPES *peach syrup (page 124).*

PLUM AND PRUNE

★ CALCIUM, IRON, MAGNESIUM, PHOSPHORUS, POTASSIUM, FIBRE, NATURAL SUGAR

● BONES AND JOINTS Gout, rheumatism.

● BLOOD AND CIRCULATION Atherosclerosis.

● DIGESTIVE SYSTEM Constipation.

Both plums and prunes are a good source of fibre – prunes are well known for their laxative effects. Prunes also aid liver function, help to lower levels of cholesterol in the blood and have anti-cancer properties.

RECIPES *spicy spinach, prunes and beans (page 101).*

MELON (ALL TYPES)

★ VITAMINS A, B, C, NATURAL SUGAR, WATER

● BONES AND JOINTS Gout, rheumatism.

● DIGESTIVE SYSTEM Constipation, dyspepsia, irritable bowel syndrome.

Melon is cooling, laxative and diuretic. Applied topically, crushed melon flesh eases the pain of mild burns, including sunburn. A beauty lotion for dry skin can be made with equal amounts of distilled water, milk and melon juice.

RECIPES *minted melon (page 106), watermelon and summer fruits (page 106).*

BLACKCURRANT

★ VITAMIN C, CALCIUM, MAGNESIUM, PHOSPHORUS, POTASSIUM, NATURAL SUGAR

● BONES AND JOINTS Gout, rheumatism.

● IMMUNE SYSTEM Sore throat.

Blackcurrants promote vitality and speed recovery after illness. They may aid bone remineralization after fractures. The leaves have the same properties as the berries and are also diuretic.

RECIPES blackcurrant wine (page 121).

REDCURRANT

★ VITAMINS A, B, C, CALCIUM, IRON, PHOSPHORUS, POTASSIUM, CITRIC ACID, PECTIN, NATURAL SUGAR

● BONES AND JOINTS Arthritis (rheumatoid), gout.

● DIGESTIVE SYSTEM Constipation.

● KIDNEYS AND BLADDER Cystitis.

Redcurrants are laxative, diuretic and depurative. They ease inflammation of the digestive tract, mild fever and liver problems. Redcurrants are very acidic and should not be eaten in excess.

RECIPES red- and whitecurrants with raspberry coulis (page 107), redcurrant, blackberry and blueberry juice (page 112).

BLACKBERRY

★ VITAMINS A , B, C, E, CALCIUM, PHOSPHORUS, POTASSIUM, NATURAL SUGAR, PECTIN, TANNIN, ESSENTIAL OIL

● DIGESTIVE SYSTEM Diarrhoea.

● IMMUNE SYSTEM Sore throat.

Blackberries are astringent, laxative, tonic and depurative. The syrup is a good remedy for diarrhoea in babies, respiratory infections and sore throats. An infusion of the leaves is a traditional gargle for acute sore throat.

RECIPES watermelon and summer fruits (page 106), fruit salad with lemon balm (page 107), redcurrant, blackberry and blueberry juice (page 112), blackberry syrup (page 125).

CHERRY

★ VITAMINS A, B, C, CALCIUM, MAGNESIUM, PHOSPHORUS, POTASSIUM, ELLAGIC ACID, NATURAL SUGAR

● BONES AND JOINTS Arthritis (rheumatoid), gout, rheumatism.

● BLOOD AND CIRCULATION Atherosclerosis, arteriosclerosis.

● KIDNEYS AND BLADDER Bladder stone, cystitis.

Cherries are diuretic, laxative, depurative; they stimulate the immune system and help to prevent infection. Cherry stem decoction can be used to treat cystitis, rheumatism and oedema.

RECIPES cherry-stem decoction (page 119), cherry-stem and apple decoction (page 120), cherry-leaf wine (page 122).

STRAWBERRY

★ VITAMINS A, B AND C, IRON, MAGNESIUM, PHOSPHORUS, SILICA, SULPHUR, NATURAL SUGAR, SALICYLIC ACID

● BONES AND JOINTS Gout.

● BLOOD AND CIRCULATION High blood pressure.

● DIGESTIVE SYSTEM Colitis, constipation, diarrhoea.

● KIDNEYS AND BLADDER Cystitis.

Strawberries are tonic, laxative and antibacterial. They enhance liver and gallbladder function. Strawberries may cause an allergic response (in the form of a rash) or exacerbate allergic dermatitis. The leaves and roots can be made into a medicinal decoction.

RECIPES carrot and strawberry salad (page 89), fruit salad with lemon balm (page 107), strawberry and raspberry juice (page 112), strawberry-leaf decoction (page 120).

RASPBERRY

★ VITAMINS A, B, C, IRON, MAGNESIUM, POTASSIUM, CITRIC, MALIC AND SALICYLIC ACIDS, NATURAL SUGAR

● BONES AND JOINTS Gout.

● DIGESTIVE SYSTEM Indigestion, vomiting.

● SKIN, HAIR AND NAILS Eczema.

Raspberries are slightly diuretic and laxative. They are good for frequent urination. Raspberry leaf infusion can facilitate labour.

RECIPES red- and whitecurrants with raspberry coulis (page 107), apple and raspberry juice (page 111), cherry and raspberry juice (page 112), strawberry and raspberry juice (page 112), raspberry vinegar (page 114).

CITRUS FRUIT

ORANGE

★ VITAMINS B, C, CALCIUM, COPPER, MANGANESE, PHOSPHORUS, POTASSIUM, ZINC, BIOFLAVONOIDS, NATURAL SUGAR, PECTIN

● DIGESTIVE SYSTEM Dyspepsia.

Oranges have tonic, diuretic and laxative properties. They stimulate the immune system, liver function and appetite.

continues on page 37

blueberry

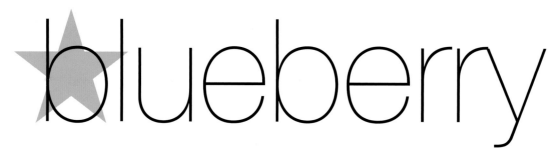

BLUEBERRIES HAVE ANTI-CANCER AND ANTIBACTERIAL PROPERTIES. THEY ARE GOOD FOR THE HEALTH OF THE EYES, INTESTINES, CIRCULATORY SYSTEM AND URINARY TRACT.

The properties of blueberry

Blueberries are part of the *Vaccinium* species, which also includes cranberries and bilberries. They are small, purple berries that are commonly found in western and central Europe and North America. Thought to have been used in European folk medicine since the 16th century, blueberries have excellent antioxidant properties which make them useful for preventing cancer and other degenerative diseases. In fact, when compared to other fruits, blueberries are among the top sources of antioxidants.

Blueberries have a powerful antibacterial action in the intestine – especially upon coli bacteria – they promote the healing of gastric ulcers, and the leaves of the blueberry plant contain tannin, which has strong anti-diarrhoeal properties.

Blood circulation is enhanced by substances found in blueberries, such as vitamins A and C, bioflavonoids, antho-cyanosides, glycosides and delphininol. Blueberries may help to lower blood sugar, decrease the chances of blood clots forming and enhance the health of blood capillaries.

Blueberries can improve eyesight. This is thought to be due to compounds in the berries that enhance the health of capillaries in the eye.

Cranberries (*Vaccinium macrocarpon*) are a close relative of blueberries and are native to North America. They are a well-known and popular treatment for urinary-tract infections, such as cystitis (an inflammation of the bladder resulting in frequent, urgent and often painful urination). Drinking the fresh juice of either blueberries or cranberries can help to prevent urinary tract infections.

Blueberries in the diet

Since blueberries are excellent antioxidants, they are important in the diet to promote long-term health and to prevent age-related physical changes and chronic diseases. In particular, people with cardiovascular problems, mild diabetes, eye problems, urinary tract or intestinal infections should eat blueberries regularly. Blueberries make wonderful pies, syrups and jam and are much enjoyed by children. They can be made into liqueurs or preserves for adults or the berries can be added to fruit salad or simply eaten as a snack on their own.

Medicinal preparations

In addition to eating blueberries, the berries and leaves can be made into medicinal preparations. Blueberry decoction is useful for diarrhoea, colitis and poor night vision. It can be used as a mouthwash for sore throats and ulcers, and as a face wash for eczema. To make, boil 75 g blueberries in 1 litre of water until the volume of water has halved. Strain and use as appropriate.

Blueberry and strawberry leaf decoction is good for mild diabetes, intestinal problems, arteriosclerosis, rheumatism and arthritis and can be drunk throughout the day. Boil 20 g each of blueberry and strawberry leaves in 1 litre of water for 3 minutes. Leave to infuse for 10 minutes, strain and drink. To make a tincture of blueberries, add 100 g fresh blueberries, a handful of blueberry leaves and the zest of one lemon to 700 ml vodka. Leave in a cool, dark place for 3 weeks and then press and strain the mixture and store in a tightly sealed bottle. Take 20–30 drops of this tincture in a glass of water every day for diarrhoea, intestinal problems, circulatory problems and mild diabetes. It can also be as a gargle for sore throats.

STAR FOOD PROFILE

- **BONES AND JOINTS** Arthritis (rheumatoid), rheumatism.

- **BLOOD AND CIRCULATION** Atherosclerosis, arteriosclerosis, Raynaud's disease.

- **DIGESTIVE SYSTEM** Abdominal cramp and colic, colitis, diarrhoea, gastroenteritis, intestinal infections, ulcerative colitis.

- **KIDNEYS AND BLADDER** Cystitis and urethritis.

- **IMMUNE SYSTEM** Sore throat.

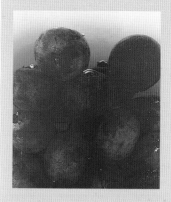

blueberry vinegar

Use in dressings or take a teaspoon, diluted in water, every morning.

300 g blueberries
700 ml white wine vinegar or cider vinegar

Put the blueberries in a hermetically-sealable pickling jar. Pour over the white-wine or cider vinegar and seal the jar tightly. Leave to macerate in a cool, dark place for 2 weeks. Strain and bottle the vinegar.

blueberries and cottage cheese

200 g cottage cheese
3 tablespoons caster sugar
3 tablespoons live yoghurt
200 g fresh blueberries
1 apple, peeled and grated
Lemon juice to taste
To garnish: a few raspberries

Beat the cottage cheese with the sugar and yoghurt. Stir in the blueberries, apple and lemon juice. Garnish with raspberries. Chill and serve.

blueberry syrup

This can be added to water for children or to white wine for adults.

1 kg blueberries
300 ml water
Sugar

In a stainless steel saucepan bring the blueberries and water to the boil. Strain them through muslin. Allow the juice to ferment at room temperature for 24 hours. Weigh the juice and add an equal amount of sugar. Dissolve the sugar in the juice, bring to the boil, simmer for 1 minute and allow to cool. Store the syrup in sterilized bottles in the refrigerator.

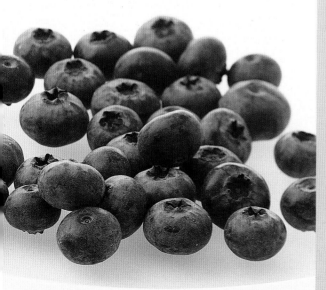

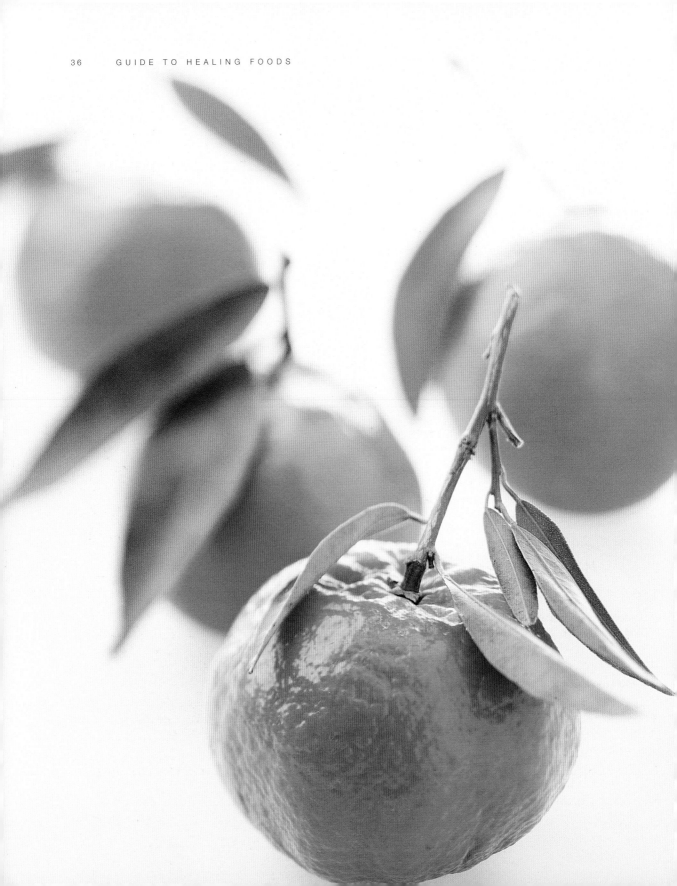

Oranges also help to lower levels of cholesterol in the blood and they are rich in antioxidants. Eating whole oranges is preferable to drinking concentrated juice.

RECIPES *radish and kumquat salad (page 90), orange-zest infusion (page 117).*

MANDARIN AND TANGERINE

★ VITAMINS B, C, CALCIUM, COPPER, MANGANESE, PHOSPHORUS, POTASSIUM, ZINC, BIOFLAVONOIDS, NATURAL SUGAR, PECTIN

Mandarin and tangerine have similar properties to orange. Mandarin rind contains an essential oil that acts as a sedative and, in Chinese medicine, an infusion of dried tangerine peel is used for poor digestion, abdominal distension and irritability.

GRAPEFRUIT

★ VITAMINS B, C, COPPER, MAGNESIUM, POTASSIUM, ANTIOXIDANTS, BIOFLAVONOIDS, ESSENTIAL OIL, NATURAL SUGAR, PECTIN

● BONES AND JOINTS Arthritis (rheumatoid).

● DIGESTIVE SYSTEM Dyspepsia, obesity.

Grapefruit has strong antioxidant and cholesterol-lowering properties. It contains an astringent essential oil, stimulates appetite and liver function, aids detoxification, and is slightly diuretic. Grapefruit is recommended for circulatory problems and obesity. It has a negative interaction with a variety of prescribed drugs – consult your doctor if in doubt.

OTHER FRUIT

APPLE

★ VITAMINS B, C, IRON, MAGNESIUM, MANGANESE, PHOSPHORUS, POTASSIUM, SULPHUR, NATURAL SUGAR, PECTIN, MALIC ACID

● BONES AND JOINTS Arthritis (rheumatoid), gout, rheumatism.

● DIGESTIVE SYSTEM Constipation, diarrhoea, dyspepsia, peptic ulcers.

Apples are gently diuretic, they aid the elimination of uric acid and lower levels of cholesterol in the blood. Traditionally, raw apples are eaten to ease constipation and cooked apples are eaten as a remedy for diarrhoea. Apple blossom infusion can ease coughs and sore throats.

RECIPES *autumn fruit compote (page 108), apple and raspberry juice (page 111), cherry and apple juice (page 112), pear and apple infusion (page 118), cherry-stem and apple decoction (page 120).*

PEAR

★ VITAMIN A, B, C, COPPER, IODINE, MAGNESIUM, PHOSPHORUS, SULPHUR, ZINC, NATURAL SUGAR, PECTIN

● BONES AND JOINTS Arthritis (rheumatoid), gout, rheumatism.

● DIGESTIVE SYSTEM Diarrhoea.

Pears are laxative, diuretic, astringent and calming. They aid uric acid elimination and prevent bacteria proliferating in the intestines. They are good for pregnant women, elderly people and convalescents. An infusion of pear tree leaves can ease urinary problems.

RECIPES *autumn fruit compote (page 108), pears with herbs (page 108), pear and apple infusion (page 118).*

PHYSALIS

★ VITAMIN C, PHYSALIN

● BONES AND JOINTS Arthritis (rheumatoid), gout.

● KIDNEYS AND BLADDER Bladder stones.

Physalis contains physalin, which is diuretic and facilitates the elimination of urea. The jam is good for kidney or bladder inflammation.

RECIPES *physalis jam (page 116), physalis-berry decoction (page 120).*

PERSIMMON

★ VITAMINS A, B, C, COPPER, IODINE, MAGNESIUM, PHOSPHORUS, SULPHUR, ZINC, NATURAL SUGAR, PECTIN

● DIGESTIVE SYSTEM Crohn's disease.

Persimmon is a nutritious fruit that prevents the proliferation of bacteria in the intestines. It has laxative and astringent properties.

POMEGRANATE

★ VITAMINS A, B, C, TRACE ELEMENTS, NATURAL SUGAR

● BLOOD AND CIRCULATION High blood pressure.

● DIGESTIVE SYSTEM Constipation.

Pomegranate is considered to be a tonic for the heart, kidneys and bladder. The juice is recommended for people with bladder disorders or tapeworm.

QUINCE

★ VITAMINS A, B, C, CALCIUM, COPPER, IRON, MAGNESIUM, PHOSPHORUS, NATURAL SUGAR, PECTIN, TANNIN

● DIGESTIVE SYSTEM Diarrhoea.

Quince has astringent properties and enhances digestion and liver function.

RECIPES *quince liqueur (page 123).*

continues on page 41

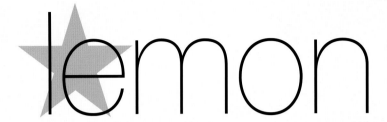
lemon

LEMON IS A NATURAL DISINFECTANT. IT IS RICH IN VITAMIN C AND CITRUS FLAVONOIDS THAT HAVE A POWERFUL ANTIOXIDANT FUNCTION. LEMON IS GOOD FOR STRENGTHENING THE IMMUNE SYSTEM AND PREVENTING INFECTION AND DISEASE.

The properties of lemon

The lemon tree *(Citrus limon)* is a small evergreen indigenous to the forests of northern India. It bears bright yellow segmented fruit that, together with lime, orange and grapefruit, belong to the citrus family (page 33).

Although there is some doubt about their origin and distribution, it is thought that lemon trees were introduced to Europe by Arabs, probably around the 11th century. In the past, lemons were the mainstay of prevention and treatment for scurvy, a disease that results from a deficiency of vitamin C. Lemons were traditionally taken on long sea voyages and the juice given to sailors in order to prevent scurvy. Today, lemons are widely produced in the USA, Spain, Portugal, Italy and, to a lesser extent, southern France.

Lemons are rich in citrus flavonoids that, alongside vitamin C, have an important antioxidant function. Citrus flavonoids are phytochemicals (biologically active plant compounds) that can assist the healing of wounds, strengthen the walls of blood capillaries and prevent diseases such as arteriosclerosis. Vitamin C also helps to fight infection, strengthen the immune system, make collagen (the main protein found in connective tissue), keep the skin and joints healthy and prevent cancer. Other substances found in lemon are citric and malic acid, vitamins A and B, glucose, fructose, potassium, phosphorus, silica, manganese and copper.

Pectin is another important component of lemon. It is concentrated in the skin around the segments and can help to lower levels of unhealthy cholesterol in the blood.

Lemon as a cure

Lemons can be used to treat a range of ailments. They are a natural booster of the immune system; they can help to reduce mild fever, lower blood pressure, reduce gastric acidity, promote liver function and increase the fluidity of blood. They also have diuretic properties.

Specific illnesses that can be treated with lemon are rheumatism, arthritis, high blood cholesterol, dyspepsia, colds and influenza. As well as using lemons in recipes, try to use the juice freely as a flavouring in cooking, as a dressing for salads and fish, and in cold drinks and teas.

Lemon juice is a natural disinfectant and antiseptic – prior to the development of modern antiseptics, it was used in hospitals for this purpose. The juice can be applied directly to the skin – it is an astringent and a bactericide – and it is a useful ingredient in home-made beauty masks. Lemon juice can be used as a skin toner, an anti-aging treatment and to reduce or eliminate freckles.

A fragrant essential oil is found in the outer skin of the lemon and this can be extracted under pressure. This essential oil has excellent anti-bacterial properties and is available from health food shops, aromatherapy suppliers and some pharmacies. It can be used to treat colds, sore throats, gingivitis or mouth ulcers. Take four drops in a teaspoon of honey for colds and sore throats. For gingivitis or mouth ulcers, use one drop of essential oil on a toothbrush with a small amount of toothpaste. This will disinfect the teeth and mouth. Lemon essential oil is also antiparasitic.

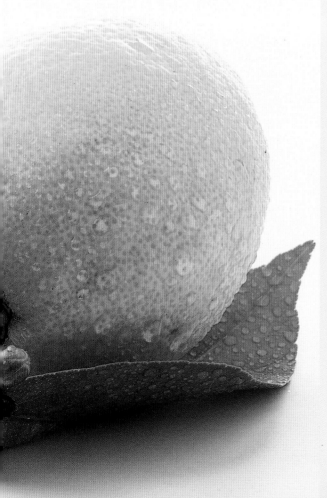

STAR FOOD PROFILE

- **BONES AND JOINTS** Arthritis (rheumatoid), rheumatism.
- **BLOOD AND CIRCULATION** Atherosclerosis, palpitations.
- **DIGESTIVE SYSTEM** Dyspepsia.
- **IMMUNE SYSTEM** Colds, influenza, sore throat.

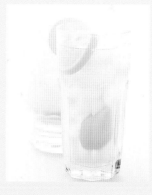

lemonade

2 lemons, wiped and sliced
60 g brown sugar
1 litre water

Mix the lemons with the water and sugar. Leave to macerate for
12 hours in the refrigerator, stirring intermittently to dissolve the sugar,
and then drink cold.

lemon preserved in salt

Use in salads or stews. The lemon juice can also be used, sparingly, as
a seasoning.

3 lemons, wiped and quartered
Salt

In a small, hermetically-sealable pickling jar, put a 1 cm-deep layer
of salt. Place one layer of lemon quarters on top and cover with salt.
Continue until the last layer of lemon is covered in salt and then tightly
seal the jar and store in a cool, dark place for 1 month. After a month,
wash the lemon quarters under cold, running water and use.

lemon in oil

Lemons will keep for months if they are covered in oil – use them in
salads or with meat or fish dishes. The oil can be used in dressings.

6 lemons, wiped and sliced or quartered
3 tablespoons salt
Olive oil
1 bay leaf

Place the lemons in a bowl and sprinkle them with the salt. Toss and
then refrigerate for 24 hours. Drain the juice from the lemons, then leave
in a colander for 2 hours, or press the lemon gently to remove as much
juice as possible. Wipe the salt off the lemons and place in a hermetically-
sealable pickling jar. Cover the lemons with the olive oil – press them
down to make sure they are covered – and add the bay leaf.

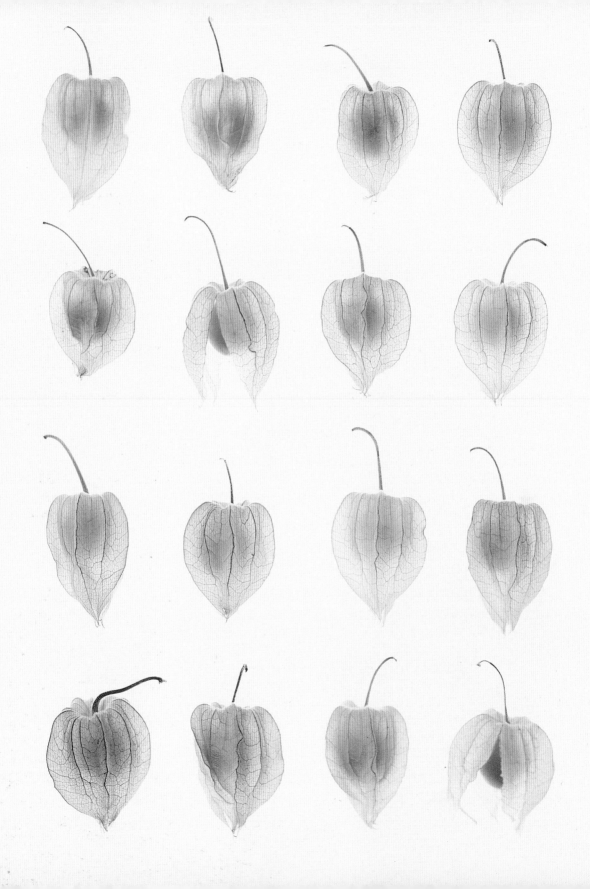

RHUBARB

★ VITAMINS B, C, IRON, MAGNESIUM

● DIGESTIVE SYSTEM Constipation.

Rhubarb has tonic, laxative and anti-parasitic properties. It facilitates bile flow and prevents the proliferation of bacteria in the gut. The root may be used in powder or tincture form as a laxative. Rhubarb should be avoided by people suffering from hyperacidity, gout, kidney stones or gallstones. The leaves are poisonous.
RECIPES *rhubarb and ginger tart (page 107).*

NUTS

HAZELNUT

★ CALCIUM, PHOSPHORUS, COPPER, IRON, MAGNESIUM, POTASSIUM, SULPHUR, POLYUNSATURATED FATTY ACIDS

Hazelnuts are excellent energy-providing snacks that are also rich in fibre. They are recommended for people who are prone to kidney or gall bladder stones. They may also help get rid of intestinal worms – treatment consists of 1 tablespoon of cold-pressed hazelnut oil every morning on an empty stomach for 15 days. Cold-pressed hazelnut oil can also be used externally. It is particularly recommended for oily skin owing to its regulatory effect on sebum secretion. It can be helpful in the treatment of acne, dermatitis and seborrhoeic eczema. An infusion of hazelnut leaves makes an excellent astringent fluid that can be applied to the skin for the treatment of varicose veins. Cover 30 g of dried leaves with 1 litre of boiling water and infuse for 12 hours – strain and use as a skin wash two or three times a day. A fluid extract from the leaves (readily available) can be taken internally for the same condition.
RECIPES *green beans with dijon mustard (page 105).*

ALMOND

★ VITAMINS A, B, CALCIUM, MAGNESIUM, PHOSPHORUS, POTASSIUM, OLEIC ACID

● DIGESTIVE SYSTEM Irritable bowel syndrome.

Almonds are an energy-providing and nutritious snack. They have a balancing effect upon the nervous system and are useful for digestive problems. Almond milk relieves intestinal spasm and inflammation in cases of irritable bowel syndrome; sweet almond oil is a mild laxative that is recommended for children. Externally, almond paste and oil can be used for eczema, rashes, and as an ingredient in beauty masks. Bitter almonds are toxic and should be avoided.
RECIPES *almond milk (page 71)*

CHESTNUT

★ VITAMINS B, C, IRON, MAGNESIUM, POTASSIUM, ZINC

● BLOOD AND CIRCULATION Anaemia.

● DIGESTIVE SYSTEM Dyspepsia.

Chestnuts are good for convalescents, elderly people and those prone to varicose veins and haemorrhoids. A handful of the leaves infused for 10 minutes in 1 litre of water is a good expectorant.
RECIPES *brussels sprouts with chestnuts (page 104).*

PINE NUT

★ VITAMINS A, B, CALCIUM, MAGNESIUM, PHOSPHORUS, POTASSIUM, ZINC, OLEIC ACID

Pine nuts are energy-providing and nutritious; they have laxative properties and can help to ease digestive problems.

PEANUT

★ VITAMINS B, E, TRACE ELEMENTS AND AMYLASE

● DIGESTIVE SYSTEM Dyspepsia.

Peanuts contain amylase, an enzyme that eases dyspepsia and hyperacidity. Some people are allergic to peanuts: the symptoms include vomiting and diarrhoea. In severe cases the allergy is fatal.

WALNUT

★ VITAMINS A, B, C, COPPER, IRON, MAGNESIUM, POTASSIUM, SELENIUM, ZINC, LINOLEIC AND OLEIC ACID

● DIGESTIVE SYSTEM Diarrhoea.

Walnuts have astringent and cholesterol-lowering properties and are good for getting rid of intestinal parasites and for alleviating heart and circulatory problems. Walnut oil can be applied to skin affected by dermatitis or eczema.
RECIPES *garlic and walnut sauce (page 49).*

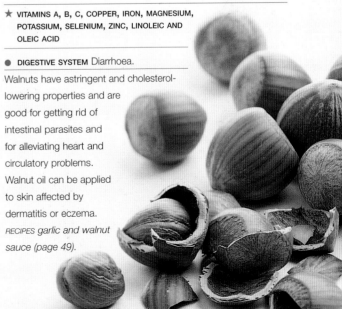

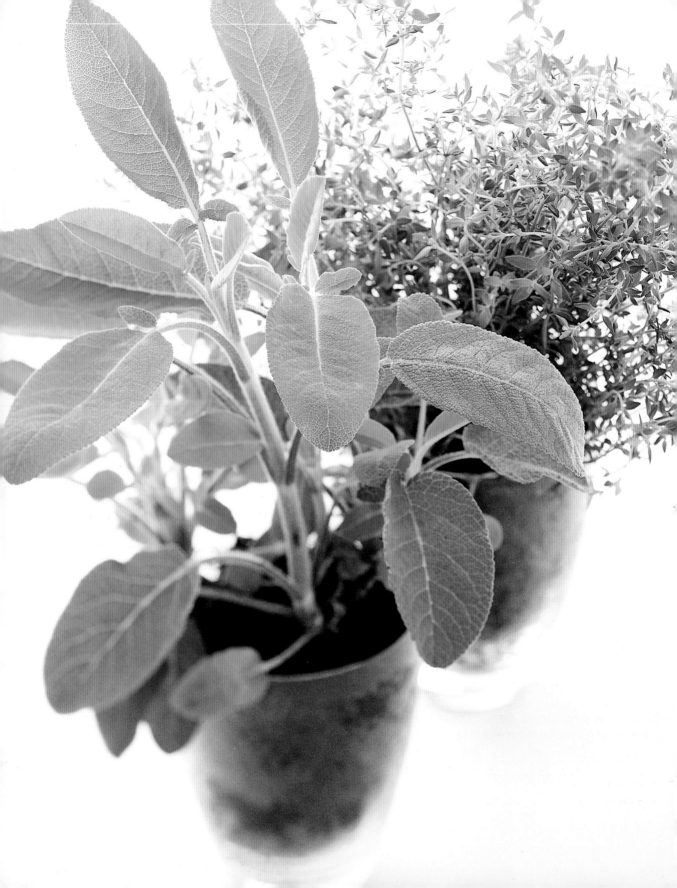

herbs, spices and condiments

HERBS

PARSLEY

★ VITAMINS A, B, C, IRON, ESSENTIAL OIL

● BLOOD AND CIRCULATION Anaemia.

● DIGESTIVE SYSTEM Dyspepsia, flatulence.

Parsley has diuretic, depurative, tonic and laxative properties. It stimulates appetite and liver function, regulates bile flow and is a good antiseptic for the lungs. Parsley is best eaten raw in salads or chopped and sprinkled generously over casseroles, meat, fish and other main-course dishes. It can also be used in broths or in raw juice cocktails. Freshly chopped parsley can be rubbed into the skin as an anti-aging treatment or as a remedy for insect bites and stings. An infusion of parsley seeds can be used to treat urine retention and digestive problems such as dyspepsia.

RECIPES *parsley, onion and lemon salad (page 93), taboule (page 94), potatoes with herb sauce (page 105).*

MINT

★ ESSENTIAL OIL

● BLOOD AND CIRCULATION Palpitations.

● DIGESTIVE SYSTEM Colic, colitis, intestinal parasites, irritable bowel syndrome, nausea and vomiting (including morning sickness).

● RESPIRATORY SYSTEM Asthma, bronchitis.

● NERVOUS SYSTEM, MIND AND EMOTIONS Mental fatigue, migraine, neuralgia.

Mint is a nervous-system stimulant (an infusion of mint taken in the evening may prevent sleep). Mint essential oil is a powerful antispasmodic, analgesic, anti-inflammatory and antiseptic agent for the intestines; it may also help to expel intestinal worms.

RECIPES *taboule (page 94), minted melon (page 106), fresh mint sorbet (page 107), mint syrup (page 125).*

BASIL

★ ESSENTIAL OIL

● BONES AND JOINTS Gout.

● DIGESTIVE SYSTEM Abdominal cramp, colic, intestinal infections.

● NERVOUS SYSTEM, MIND AND EMOTIONS Anxiety, insomnia, mental fatigue, migraine.

Basil is a popular herb in Mediterranean countries. It contains a powerful essential oil that has antispasmodic and antiseptic properties; it acts as a tonic for the nervous system and helps to ease digestive complaints, including intestinal infections. Basil can be used in soups, sauces, medicinal drinks, such as basil liqueur, or raw in salads. Fresh basil leaves can be preserved by freezing or storing in oil. To preserve basil in oil, choose leaves from the top part of the plant, rinse gently in cold water and allow to dry on kitchen paper. Sprinkle the leaves with salt, wait 30 minutes, gently wipe the salt off, place the leaves in a sterilized jar or bottle and fill with cold-pressed olive oil. Keep the jar tightly closed and store in the refrigerator.

RECIPES *polenta with basil tomato sauce (page 99), pasta twists with pesto (page 98), basil liqueur (page 123).*

MARJORAM AND OREGANO

★ ESSENTIAL OIL

● DIGESTIVE SYSTEM Abdominal pain, distention and wind.

● RESPIRATORY SYSTEM Bronchitis, colds, influenza.

Marjoram and oregano are two distinct plants, but for culinary and medicinal purposes they are interchangeable. Both are potent bactericides, expectorants and digestive-system stimulants. They are good natural remedies for ear, nose, throat and lung infections. The essential oils of these herbs can be applied to the skin as a treatment for rheumatism and skin infections. They should be diluted with a base oil, such as almond, before they are applied to the skin.

RECIPES *marjoram infusion (page 117).*

ROSEMARY

★ ESSENTIAL OIL

● BONES AND JOINTS Gout.

● DIGESTIVE SYSTEM Colitis, diarrhoea, flatulence, intestinal infections, irritable bowel syndrome.

● RESPIRATORY SYSTEM Asthma.

● NERVOUS SYSTEM, MIND AND EMOTIONS Headache, neuralgia.

● IMMUNE SYSTEM Colds, influenza.

Rosemary contains a potent essential oil that is diuretic, promotes perspiration, stimulates the production and flow of bile, improves digestion and acts as an antiseptic for the lungs and the digestive system. It can be diluted with a base oil, such as almond, then massaged into the skin to ease muscular cramps or rheumatism.

RECIPES carrots with rosemary (page 15).

THYME

★ ESSENTIAL OIL

● BONES AND JOINTS Rheumatis.

● DIGESTIVE SYSTEM Intestinal infections and parasites.

● RESPIRATORY SYSTEM Bronchitis, cough.

● KIDNEYS AND BLADDER Cystitis.

● IMMUNE SYSTEM Colds, influenza.

Thyme has powerful antibacterial properties. It is a general stimulant and acts as an antiseptic for the throat, lungs and digestive system. Thyme may improve poor circulation.

RECIPES amazingly aromatic vinegar (page 116).

TARRAGON

★ ESSENTIAL OIL

● DIGESTIVE SYSTEM Colic, intestinal parasites.

● WOMEN'S HEALTH Period pain.

Tarragon is a general stimulant, it is antispasmodic and improves digestive function. The infused oil can be applied to the skin to treat rheumatism, muscular spasms and cramps. Fill a jar with tarragon leaves, cover with olive oil and leave for two weeks.

RECIPES tarragon vinegar (page 116), amazingly aromatic vinegar (page 116).

SAGE

★ ESSENTIAL OIL

● WOMEN'S HEALTH Irregular or painful periods, menopausal symptoms.

There are more than 200 species of sage but the one most commonly used in cooking is Salvia officinalis. Sage is a general stimulant and a digestive-system tonic. It is good for hypotension, excessive perspiration and fatigue.

RECIPES garlic and sage soup (page 49).

BAY

★ ESSENTIAL OIL

● DIGESTIVE SYSTEM Cyspepsia, flatulence.

● WOMEN'S HEALTH Period pain.

Bay leaves have antiseptic, stimulant and antispasmodic properties. They can be used in casseroles and soups or made into an infusion for indigestion and bloated stomach, or as a gargle for mouth and throat infections (add 3–4 leaves to a cup of boiling water, cover, infuse for 10 minutes and then strain).

RECIPES orange-zest infusion (page 117).

CHIVE AND SPRING ONION

★ VITAMINS A, B, C, CALCIUM, MAGNESIUM, PHOSPHORUS, POTASSIUM, SULPHUR COMPOUNDS, BIOFLAVONOIDS, ESSENTIAL OIL

● BONES AND JOINTS Arthritis (rheumatoid), gout, rheumatism.

● BLOOD AND CIRCULATION Arteriosclerosis.

● DIGESTIVE SYSTEM Diabetes, diarrhoea, intestinal infections and parasites.

● WOMEN'S HEALTH Period pain.

Chives and spring onions are antibacterial, antiviral, antifungal and diuretic; they prevent tumour and blood-clot formation and help to lower levels of cholesterol in the body. Chives and spring onions also prevent water retention, promote the elimination of urea and the expectoration of mucus and are good for the digestive and circulatory systems. Both chives and spring onions may be eaten raw, chopped and sprinkled over main courses and salads, or made into raw juice cocktails. A broth containing chives or spring onions (especially combined with garlic, clove and ginger) can alleviate colds and influenza as well as digestive problems, such as diarrhoea. The fresh juice can be applied to insect stings, warts and boils.

RECIPES chive and ginger broth (page 88), leek and chive mimosa with polenta (page 99).

CORIANDER

★ VITAMIN B, FOLIC ACID, ESSENTIAL OIL

- ● **DIGESTIVE SYSTEM** Abdominal pain, dyspepsia, flatulence, indigestion, irritable bowel syndrome.

Coriander is an aromatic herb that has antibiotic properties and helps to treat a range of digestive problems. It is widely used in Asian and North African cooking. The leaves can be chopped and sprinkled on salads, main dishes and soups. The seeds contain a greater concentration of active ingredients than the leaves and can be made into medicinal drinks.

RECIPES coriander dressing (page 89), coriander-seed infusion (page 119), coriander-seed tincture (page 124).

CHERVIL

- ★ **VITAMINS A, B, C, IRON, ESSENTIAL OIL**
- ● **BONES AND JOINTS** Gout.
- ● **BLOOD AND CIRCULATION** Anaemia.
- ● **RESPIRATORY SYSTEM** Bronchitis.

Chervil has diuretic, tonic and laxative properties. It stimulates appetite and liver function and regulates the flow of bile. It is also a good antiseptic for the lungs and helps to get rid of phlegm in the chest. Chervil can be eaten raw in salad or sprinkled generously over casseroles, fish, meat and main course dishes. It can also be used in broths or raw juice cocktails. Freshly chopped chervil can also be rubbed on the skin to treat insect bites or stings.

RECIPES herbal broth (page 86), parsley, onion and lemon salad (page 93), potatoes with herb sauce (page 105).

BORAGE

- ★ **GAMMA-LINOLENIC ACID**
- ● **RESPIRATORY SYSTEM** Bronchitis.

Borage has depurative, diuretic and laxative properties and promotes the elimination of toxins. Borage seeds contain gama-linoleic acid (GLA), an essential fatty acid that helps the body to make prostaglandins. Prostaglandins are hormone-like substances that have numerous health benefits, such as keeping the blood thin, lowering blood pressure, maintaining water balance and regulating blood sugar. Another good, but less abundant source of GLA is evening primrose oil. Borage oil can be applied to the skin as a treatment for mature skin and dry, scaly eczema. Young borage leaves are excellent raw in salads, especially with dandelion and watercress. They can also be added to soups or included in a variety of raw juice cocktails.

RECIPES borage leaves in vinegar (page 116).

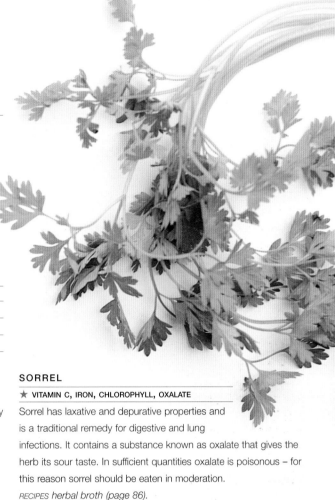

SORREL

- ★ **VITAMIN C, IRON, CHLOROPHYLL, OXALATE**

Sorrel has laxative and depurative properties and is a traditional remedy for digestive and lung infections. It contains a substance known as oxalate that gives the herb its sour taste. In sufficient quantities oxalate is poisonous – for this reason sorrel should be eaten in moderation.

RECIPES herbal broth (page 86).

SAVORY

- ★ **ESSENTIAL OIL**
- ● **DIGESTIVE SYSTEM** Diarrhoea, flatulence.
- ● **RESPIRATORY SYSTEM** Asthma, bronchitis.

Two species of savory are commonly used in cooking: summer savory (usually grown in the garden), and winter savory (usually found in the wild). Savory is a nervous system stimulant and a tonic. It is particularly effective for poor digestion.

CAMOMILE

- ★ **COMPLEX CHEMICALS SUCH AS NOBILINE AND CHAMAZULENE, ESSENTIAL OIL**
- ● **DIGESTIVE SYSTEM** Colic, diarrhoea, indigestion, irritable bowel syndrome.
- ● **NERVOUS SYSTEM, MIND AND EMOTIONS** Insomnia, migraine, neuralgia.
- ● **WOMEN'S HEALTH** Period pain.

Camomile contains nobiline, which is a bitter tonic, and also chamazulene, a potent anti-inflammatory agent. An infusion of camomile is widely recommended for its calming properties and its ability to improve digestion and ease digestive problems. Camomile infusion stimulates liver function and regulates the flow of bile. It can be used externally as a douche for thrush, a wash for inflamed skin, mild burns, sunburn, dermatitis and eczema, and as an eyewash for conjunctivitis. Camomile flowers mixed with white wine is an excellent bitter aperitif.

RECIPES lemon-balm and camomile infusion (page 118), elder and camomile infusion (page 118), camomile and citrus wine (page 123), camomile aperitif (page 123).

ELDER

★ ESSENTIAL OIL

Elderflowers promote perspiration (useful for colds and influenza) and help to advance skin eruptions in chicken pox, German measles and scarlet fever. They are diuretic, promote detoxification and stimulate bile flow. Elderberries ease constipation, headache and mild neuralgia. The bark, which is diuretic, is useful for rheumatism, arthritis, nephritis (inflammation of the kidneys) and bladder stones. All parts of the elder plant have anti-inflammatory properties.

RECIPES elder and camomile infusion (page 118), elderberry syrup (page 125).

LINDEN (LIME TREE)

★ ESSENTIAL OIL

Linden- or lime-tree blossom has antispasmodic, sedative and slight hypnotic properties. It also induces sweating. Research suggests that lime flowers may reduce the viscosity and rate of coagulation of the blood. This may help to prevent cardiovascular problems. An infusion of lime blossom has a delicate fragrance and is a good remedy for insomnia in children as well as adults (steep a small handful of the blossom in 300 ml water for 5 minutes).

RECIPES pears with herbs (page 108).

LEMON BALM (MELISSA)

★ ESSENTIAL OIL

● **DIGESTIVE SYSTEM** Indigestion.

● **NERVOUS SYSTEM, MIND AND EMOTIONS** Anxiety, insomnia, migraine, neuralgia.

Lemon balm contains a potent essential oil that has tonic and antispasmodic properties. Although rarely used in cooking, lemon balm is often included in herbal liqueurs such as Chartreuse, Benedictine and Eau de Melissa des Carmes. Lemon balm can help to relieve spasms (muscular, digestive or asthmatic).

RECIPES lemon-balm and camomile infusion (page 118), sparkling lemon-balm infusion (page 119).

DILL

★ ESSENTIAL OIL

● **DIGESTIVE SYSTEM** Abdominal cramp, colic.

● **WOMEN'S HEALTH** Irregular periods, period pain.

Dill is a type of wild fennel that is often used in fish recipes or in pickling vinegar. Both the leaves and the seeds can be used. Dill is recommended for lactating mothers as its aromatic compounds pass into breast milk and enhance the flavour.

RECIPES red lentil soup (page 89), dill-seed decoction (page 120), amazingly aromatic vinegar (page 116).

SPICES AND SEEDS

CHILLI

★ VITAMIN C, TRACE ELEMENTS, ESSENTIAL OIL CONTAINING UP TO 1% CAPSAICIN

● **DIGESTIVE SYSTEM** Diarrhoea, dyspepsia, flatulence.

● **IMMUNE SYSTEM** Colds.

There may be over 50 species of chilli of varying shapes and sizes. The colour of a chilli – green, yellow, red or purple – indicates its stage of maturity. An essential oil in chillies contains capsaicin, which is thought to be good for the heart and circulation. Chillies are recommended for digestive problems and circulatory problems such as chilblains. Excessive consumption of chillies should be avoided as it may cause chronic inflammation of the stomach and intestines.

RECIPES cardamom hot sauce (page 105).

CARDAMOM

★ ESSENTIAL OIL

● **DIGESTIVE SYSTEM** Diarrhoea.

Cardamom seeds are strongly aromatic and are widely used in Indian cooking to flavour curries, sweets and desserts. They

continues on page 50

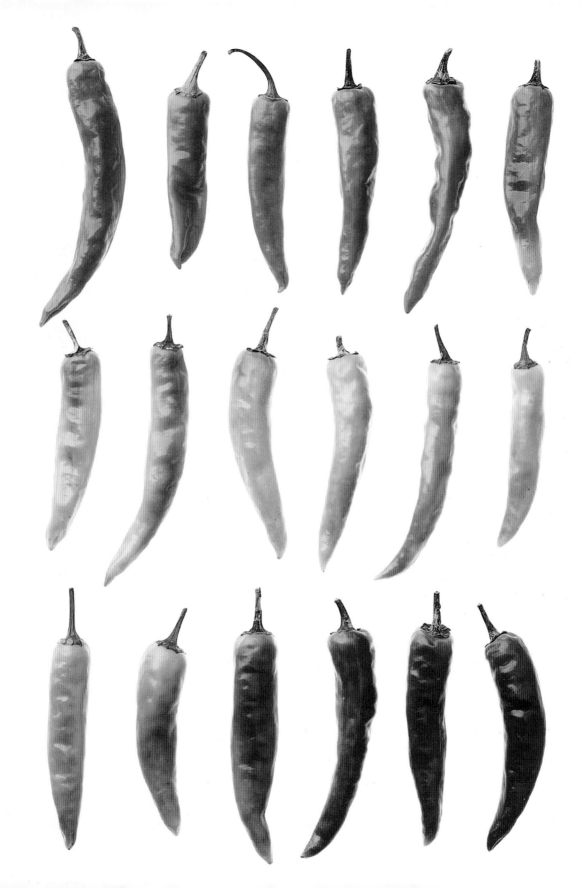

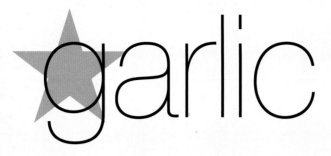

garlic

GARLIC IS AN ANTI-COAGULANT AND HELPS TO REDUCE CHOLESTEROL LEVELS IN THE BLOOD. IT ALSO HAS ANTI-BACTERIAL AND ANTI-FUNGAL PROPERTIES.

The history of garlic

Garlic is part of the Liliacaea family, which also includes onions, shallots, leeks, chives and spring onions. It is native to central Asia, and its cultivation began in China, Mesopotamia (modern Turkey, Iran and Iraq) and Egypt thousands of years ago. Garlic has a long reputation as a health-giving food used both to prevent and to cure illness. In Egypt, as early as 2600 BCE, workers building the pyramids were given garlic to keep them strong. Ancient Greek soldiers ate it to improve their strength and increase their resistance to infection. In Europe, garlic has long been used to protect against disease – 16th-century monks took it to ward off the plague and its use was widespread during the cholera epidemics of the 19th century.

The properties of garlic

The principal active ingredients in garlic are a volatile oil called allicin, released when the cloves are crushed, and several sulphur compounds, released when garlic is steamed or boiled.

Recent scientific research has shown that allicin is a powerful anti-coagulant. It inhibits blood-clotting and helps to break down existing clots, allowing the blood to flow more freely thus reducing blood pressure. Garlic inhibits the production of cholesterol in the liver and increases the rate at which dietary cholesterol is expelled from the body. As a result, it is extremely useful for those who suffer from high cholesterol levels, thrombosis (obstructive blood clots), heart disease and other circulatory problems.

Allicin has potent anti-bacterial and anti-fungal properties, and raw garlic is effective in relieving the symptoms of colds and respiratory infections, such as nasal congestion. It is also useful in combating digestive system infections and controlling the balance of bacteria in the gut, as well as helping to repel parasites, such as intestinal worms. Boiling a head of garlic in milk and drinking the resulting decoction every morning is a traditional remedy for intestinal parasites.

Recent research has suggested that diallyl sulfide, a component of garlic, may help to prevent the growth of some malignant tumours.

Garlic as a cure

A traditional European folk custom involved placing a head of garlic in a small bag and tying it around a child's neck as a protection against colds or flu. Fixing the bag around the abdomen was thought to protect against worms. Scientists have now discovered that some of the sulphur compounds found in garlic can indeed be absorbed through the skin.

For maximum therapeutic value, at least two raw garlic cloves should be eaten every day. For many people, however, this is unpalatable: odourless garlic supplements can provide a useful additional source of this important food. If you are worried about bad breath, try chewing cardamom seeds, parsley leaves or a few roasted coffee beans to help disguise the smell.

Garlic can also be used to great effect in tinctures, drinks, soups and sauces. To make a garlic tincture, soak 50 g of garlic in 250 ml of strong vodka; leave it to macerate in a sealed opaque bottle for two weeks. Strain the mixture, pressing the garlic with the back of a spoon to extract all the remaining liquid. Add up to 15 drops to a small amount of water and take twice a day to reduce high blood pressure and high cholesterol, to combat colds and chronic bronchitis or as an antiseptic for the digestive system. If you keep the tincture in an airtight bottle, away from light, it will last for up to two years.

STAR FOOD PROFILE

- **BLOOD AND CIRCULATION** Atherosclerosis, high blood pressure, thrombosis.

- **DIGESTIVE SYSTEM** Gastroenteritis, intestinal parasites, ulcerative colitis.

- **IMMUNE SYSTEM** Colds, influenza.

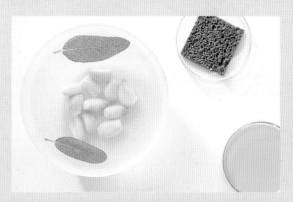

garlic and sage soup

4–5 garlic bulbs, peeled
2 litres water
Approximately 10 sage leaves
Salt and pepper
3 or 4 thick slices of rye bread
150 ml cold-pressed olive oil
To serve: fresh parsley or chervil, finely chopped

Peel the cloves from the bulbs of garlic and boil in the water for 20 minutes. Add the sage and season with salt and pepper. Leave to infuse for a few minutes. Place the rye bread in a large dish, and pour the olive oil over the bread. Pour the garlic and sage soup over the bread. Sprinkle with the parsley or chervil and serve immediately.

garlic, carrot and spinach cocktail

4 medium-sized carrots, peeled and chopped
120 g fresh spinach leaves
2 cloves of garlic, peeled
Crushed ice
Salt and pepper

Process all the ingredients in a juicer and mix with some crushed ice. Add salt and pepper to taste. Serve immediately.

garlic and walnut sauce

50 g garlic cloves, peeled
75 g shelled walnuts
250 ml walnut oil
Salt and pepper
1 tablespoon finely chopped parsley

Process all the ingredients in a blender, adding iced water if necessary.

stimulate the appetite and aid digestion. They contain an essential oil that is an effective breath freshener: after eating an excessive amount of garlic chewing cardamom seeds will both freshen the breath and prevent heartburn.

RECIPES cardamom hot sauce (page 105), poached apricots with cardamom (page 109).

CINNAMON

★ ESSENTIAL OIL

● IMMUNE SYSTEM Colds, influenza.

Cinnamon is a bactericide that improves the function of the respiratory and cardiovascular systems. It is also antispasmodic and stimulates digestion. Chinese herbalists use cinnamon to promote vitality, warm the body and treat colds and influenza.

RECIPES cinnamon wine (page 121).

CLOVES

★ ESSENTIAL OIL

● DIGESTIVE SYSTEM Diarrhoea.

● IMMUNE SYSTEM Colds, influenza.

Clove essential oil acts as a powerful antiseptic. Cloves are good for intestinal infections – travellers used to chew them in order to prevent both intestinal infections and hepatitis. They also have a slight anaesthetic action. Clove oil can be used externally to treat infected wounds, dental pain and mouth ulcers.

GINGER

★ ESSENTIAL OIL

● DIGESTIVE SYSTEM Nausea and vomiting.

● IMMUNE SYSTEM Colds, influenza.

● WOMEN'S HEALTH Morning sickness.

Ginger is one of the most widely used spices in Asia. It stimulates the appetite, has antiseptic and tonic properties and alleviates nausea, particularly morning sickness. Combined in a broth with spring onions, garlic and cloves, it promotes sweating and eases cold symptoms. Ginger can also be used as a massage oil for rheumatism or to improve blood circulation in muscles. Mix together 3 ml ginger essential oil, 1 ml rosemary essential oil, 1 ml juniper-berry essential oil and 100 ml vegetable oil.

RECIPES honey and ginger grilled salmon (page 57), chive and ginger broth (page 88), rhubarb and ginger tart (page 107), baked papaya with ginger (page 109), ginger infusion (page 119).

CUMIN

★ ESSENTIAL OIL

● DIGESTIVE SYSTEM Flatulence.

Cumin seeds are rich in an essential oil that has sedative and carminative properties. They can help to treat poor digestion and are recommended for lactating mothers.

RECIPES cumin-seed decoction (page 120).

SAFFRON

★ BITTER COMPOUNDS, ESSENTIAL OIL

● DIGESTIVE SYSTEM Dyspepsia.

● WOMEN'S HEALTH Period pain.

Saffron has calming and antispasmodic properties. It can be used to treat bronchial spasms. It can also be applied to sore and inflamed gums as a painkiller.

HORSERADISH

★ VITAMIN C, CALCIUM, IRON, MAGNESIUM, PHOSPHORUS, POTASSIUM, SULPHUR, ESSENTIAL OIL

● BONES AND JOINTS Arthritis (rheumatoid), gout, rheumatism.

● RESPIRATORY SYSTEM Bronchitis, colds, coughs.

Horseradish has antispasmodic properties, promotes the flow of bile and is good for sinus problems.

RECIPES horseradish sauce (page 105).

ANISE

★ ESSENTIAL OIL

● DIGESTIVE SYSTEM Colic, distention and wind, dyspepsia, flatulence, nausea and vomiting.

● NERVOUS SYSTEM, MIND AND EMOTIONS Migraine.

● WOMEN'S HEALTH Period pain, irregular periods.

Aniseed (the seeds of the anise plant) and star anise (the fruit) have the same properties. They both contain a potent essential oil that is strongly antispasmodic and acts as a stimulant to the heart, respiratory and digestive systems. Anise is slightly diuretic and helps to promote bile flow and digestion. It is recommended for lactating mothers.

RECIPES pears with herbs (page 108), anisette (page 123), aniseed tincture (page 124).

JUNIPER BERRIES

★ ESSENTIAL OIL

● BONES AND JOINTS Gout, rheumatism.

● **DIGESTIVE SYSTEM** Intestinal infections.

● **KIDNEYS AND BLADDER** Cystitis.

Juniper berries have tonic, antiseptic, depurative and diuretic qualities. They help to eliminate uric acid and toxins from the body and contain a powerful antibacterial essential oil. In France and neighbouring countries, houses and stables are traditionally fumigated by burning juniper twigs and leaves – their disinfectant action helps to eliminate parasites and insects. Juniper berries are good for poor digestion and chest infections; they are also recommended for diabetes because they stimulate the pancreas (the organ that produces insulin). To treat acne, eczema and slow healing wounds: boil 50 g juniper berries and twigs in 1 litre of water for 10 minutes; strain and use the cooled water as a skin wash.

RECIPES pickled turnips (page 114), juniper-berry wine (page 122).

NUTMEG

★ **ESSENTIAL OIL**

● **DIGESTIVE SYSTEM** Diarrhoea.

Nutmeg contains a potent essential oil that is poisonous in large doses, but beneficial in small amounts. It is a good general antiseptic for the digestive system, has analgesic properties and stimulates the brain and nervous system. Nutmeg is recommended for bad breath, poor digestion and other digestive ailments. The diluted essential oil can be applied to the skin for rheumatism and neuralgia (dilute with a base oil such as almond).

VANILLA

★ **ESSENTIAL OIL**

Vanilla is a mild excitant and a tonic. It also stimulates the digestive system. Vanilla essential oil has antiseptic qualities.

COCOA

★ **IRON, MAGNESIUM, THEOBROMINE, VEGETABLE FAT**

Cocoa contains theobromine, a substance that has a similar effect to caffeine, but is less toxic, does not raise blood pressure, accumulate in the body or result in addiction. Good-quality cocoa is slightly diuretic and helps to eliminate toxins from the body. In some cases, cocoa may trigger migraines. Good brands of chocolate contain at least 60 per cent cocoa.

SUNFLOWER SEED

★ **LINOLEIC, STEARIC AND PALMITIC ACIDS, POLYUNSATURATED OILS**

● **DIGESTIVE SYSTEM** Constipation.

Sunflower seeds are a useful part of a low-cholesterol diet. They are delicious toasted and provide essential fatty acids.

FENNEL SEED

★ **ESSENTIAL OILS**

● **BONES AND JOINTS** Gout.

● **DIGESTIVE SYSTEM** Abdominal pain, colic, nausea and vomiting (including morning sickness).

Fennel seeds are gently tonic and diuretic. They have an oestrogen-like effect and can help to regulate menstruation. The main medicinal use of fennel seeds is for digestive problems, such as poor appetite and digestion, bloating, nausea and flatulence. The seeds also promote urination and the elimination of uric acid.

RECIPES fennel-seed decoction (page 120).

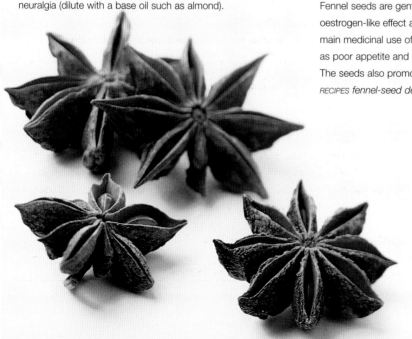

CONDIMENTS, HONEY AND WINE

PEPPERCORNS

★ TRACE ELEMENTS (INCLUDING CHROMIUM), COMPLEX ESSENTIAL OIL (PIPERIN)

● DIGESTIVE SYSTEM Diarrhoea, dyspepsia.

● IMMUNE SYSTEM Colds, sore throat.

Peppercorns are good for digestive problems and circulatory problems, such as chilblains. They stimulate the heart and peripheral circulation, although excessive consumption of pepper may aggravate any inflammation of the stomach and intestines.

VINEGAR

★ POTASSIUM, PHOSPHORUS, TRACE ELEMENTS SUCH AS COPPER AND ZINC

● BONES AND JOINTS Arthritis (rheumatoid), gout, rheumatism.

● IMMUNE SYSTEM Sore throat.

Vinegar is helpful for a variety of conditions. A gargle made of honey, vinegar and water may help to ease sore throats. Vinegar is also a traditional toner and disinfectant for the skin. Because it acts as a solvent it is able to take up the active ingredients of the medicinal plants that are preserved in it. Home-made aromatic vinegar can be added to salads or used in cooking, thereby increasing the medicinal value of other foods. Excessive consumption of vinegar should be avoided as it may upset the stomach and cause digestive problems, such as gastritis.

RECIPES *pickled turnips (page 114), pickled beetroot (page 114), pickled cauliflower (page 114), blackberry vinegar (page 114), raspberry vinegar (page 114), borage leaves in vinegar (page 116), tarragon vinegar (page 116), shallot vinegar (page 116), herb vinegar (page 116), amazingly aromatic vinegar (page 116).*

MUSTARD

★ ESSENTIAL OIL, FERMENTING AGENTS

● DIGESTIVE SYSTEM Constipation.

The white mustard seed is used as a condiment and the black seed is commonly used by herbalists. Mustard causes a sensation of heat in the stomach and stimulates the digestion.

RECIPES *table mustard (page 116).*

HONEY

★ AROMATIC SUBSTANCES, FRUCTOSE, GLUCOSE, POLLEN

● DIGESTIVE SYSTEM Diarrhoea.

● RESPIRATORY SYSTEM Asthma, bronchitis.

● IMMUNE SYSTEM Sore throat.

Honey is a natural antibiotic that works both internally and externally. It eases respiratory infections, calms the nerves, induces sleep and disinfects wounds and sores. As well as being an effective treatment for diarrhoea, it also has laxative properties. A few drops of lemon juice mixed with a teaspoon of honey is an excellent sore throat remedy.

RECIPES *honey and ginger grilled salmon (page 57), peach syrup (page 124).*

POLLEN

★ VITAMINS B, D, E, MAGNESIUM, POTASSIUM, TRACE ELEMENTS, ESSENTIAL AMINO ACIDS

Pollen is an easily assimilated natural food supplement that is recommended for anyone suffering from low energy levels. One tablespoon a day is the standard recommended dose, although some specialists recommend more.

ROYAL JELLY

★ VITAMINS B COMPLEX, C, AMINO ACIDS

● BLOOD AND CIRCULATION Anaemia.

● NERVOUS SYSTEM, MIND AND EMOTIONS Depression, mental fatigue.

Royal jelly is a white substance produced by bees to feed to the larvae of potential queen bees. It is a powerful tonic that is particularly recommended for children and elderly people.

WINE

★ BIOFLAVONOIDS, TANNINS

● BLOOD AND CIRCULATION High blood pressure.

Small amounts of wine (no more than 2 glasses a day) are recommended for enhancing the health of the cardiovascular system. Red wine, in particular, has been found to reduce the incidence of heart disease, particularly among those suffering from high cholesterol and high blood pressure.

RECIPES *blackcurrant wine (page 121), cinnamon wine (page 121), artichoke-leaf wine (page 122), cherry-leaf wine (page 122), juniper-berry wine (page 122), camomile and citrus wine (page 123), camomile aperitif (page 123).*

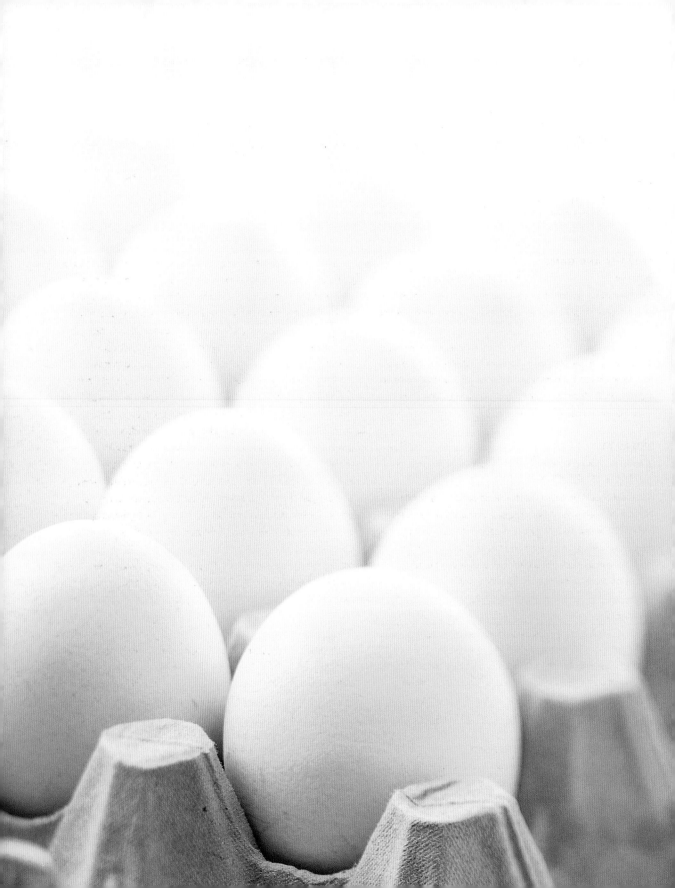

meat, fish and dairy produce

POULTRY AND GAME

★ VITAMIN B COMPLEX, IRON, TRACE ELEMENTS, ZINC, PROTEIN

The main advantage of poultry and game is that they are usually leaner than other types of meat. Red meat, for example, contains a large amount of hidden fat – this can have an adverse effect on cholesterol levels and increase the risk of fatty deposits building up in the arteries. Reducing your intake of red meat and eating game and poultry instead can reduce the risk of cardiovascular disease.
RECIPES chicken breasts with celeriac mash (page 100), chicken, millet, barley and celeriac pilaff (page 101).

RED MEAT

★ VITAMIN B COMPLEX (ESPECIALLY B12), IRON, SELENIUM, ZINC, ESSENTIAL AMINO ACIDS AND PROTEIN

Red meat should be eaten in moderation because of its high fat content. Lean cuts of lamb, pork and beef should be selected and visible fat trimmed off. Modern food production methods mean that there may be traces of antibiotics and hormones in meat. As with all food, use organic produce where possible.
RECIPES lamb with spinach and lentils (page 99).

SHELLFISH

★ IODINE, IRON, SELENIUM, ZINC AND OTHER TRACE ELEMENTS AND PROTEIN

Shellfish provide energy and are a good source of the antioxidant minerals zinc and selenium. They help to boost the immune system and are a low-fat source of protein. It is a good idea to eat shellfish on a regular basis as an alternative to meat.

MILK, CHEESE, BUTTER, YOGHURT

★ VITAMINS A, B, D, CALCIUM, ALL ESSENTIAL AMINO ACIDS, PROTEIN

Although milk and milk products are good sources of protein and calcium, they are also difficult to digest. This is because during the sterilization process milk is subjected to intense heat that destroys its natural ferments. These ferments help the digestion of lactose – the sugar found in milk. Without the aid of these bacteria, lactose intolerance becomes more likely. Symptoms of lactose intolerance include diarrhoea, bloating, abdominal pain and wind. Milk can also exacerbate eczema and respiratory problems involving mucus. If you suspect that you suffer from lactose intolerance, eliminate milk and milk products from your diet for two weeks and see if your symptoms diminish in frequency or intensity. Cheese, butter and cream should be consumed only in small quantities because they are rich in saturated fat and can contribute to the build up of fatty deposits in the arteries. Avoid these foods altogether if you are overweight or have high cholesterol levels (or switch to low-fat products). Live yoghurt is good for the health of the digestive tract and retains the natural bacteria that help to digest lactose. Dairy products can be made more digestible by mixing them with live yoghurt. For example, mix cottage cheese with 2–3 tablespoons of live yoghurt.
RECIPES cottage cheese with watercress (page 95), halibut steak and nettle butter (page 101), fresh figs with raspberry cheese (page 109).

EGG

★ VITAMINS B, D, CALCIUM, CHROMIUM, IODINE, IRON, SELENIUM, ZINC, CHOLESTEROL, PROTEIN

Eggs are a good source of protein but they should be avoided by people with high cholesterol levels. Choose organically produced free-range eggs.
RECIPES buckwheat with leek sauce (page 97), leek and chive mimosa with polenta (page 99).

oily fish
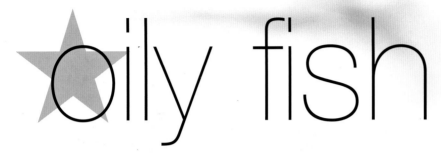

OILY FISH, SUCH AS MACKEREL, SALMON, HERRING AND TUNA, ARE
RICH IN POLYUNSATURATED FATS KNOWN AS OMEGA-3 FATTY ACIDS. A
SUBSTANTIAL BODY OF RESEARCH HAS LINKED DIETS RICH IN OMEGA-
3 FATTY ACIDS WITH A LOW INCIDENCE OF CARDIOVASCULAR DISEASE.

The properties of oily fish

Both freshwater and saltwater oily fish are an important part of
a nutritious, medicinal diet. Most nutrition experts suggest that
they should be eaten frequently, particularly as an alternative to
red meat. Oily fish are rich in vitamin D and omega-3 fatty acids
which makes them good for the health of the cardiovascular
system. Research shows that the incidence of cardiovascular
disease is lowest in populations that eat a diet high in omega-3
fatty acids – the Eskimo population, whose diet is dominated
by oily fish, is an excellent example of this.

Preventing illness

Oily fish can help to reduce some major health problems, such
as high blood pressure, atherosclerosis and arteriosclerosis. It
is estimated that regular consumption of fish and fish oil can
reduce the risk of heart attack by approximately one third. Oily
fish have an anti-inflammatory action that makes them useful
for health problems, such as ulcerative colitis and rheumatoid
arthritis, that are characterized by inflammation. Oily fish are
also recommended for eczema, psoriasis, multiple sclerosis
and they may help to protect the body from cancer. Research
suggests that omega-3 fatty acids may counteract certain
types of allergies and assist brain development in children.

An important role of omega-3 fatty acids is the creation of
prostaglandins. Prostaglandins are hormone-like substances
that have numerous health benefits, such as keeping the blood
thin, lowering blood pressure, maintaining water balance and
regulating blood sugar.

Including fish in the diet

Omega-3 fatty acids are found in a range of fish and shellfish
but the most abundant sources are mackerel, herring,
anchovies, trout, salmon, sardine, whitebait, pilchards and red
tuna. People who have had a heart attack or who suffer from
chronic cardiovascular illness are advised to eat 30 g of these
types of oily fish every day. Those who are in reasonable health
and do not have cardiovascular disease are advised to eat oily
fish twice weekly in order to maintain long-term health.

It is easy to confuse fish oil and omega-3 fatty acids with
cod liver oil. Many people take cod liver oil in supplement form
during the winter months (care should be taken as overdosing
on this may damage your health). Although cod liver oil is an
excellent source of the fat-soluble vitamins A and D, it is a poor
source of omega-3 fatty acids. The best source of omega-3
fatty acids is fresh oily fish; if this is not available, canned
sardine or mackerel is a good alternative.

STAR FOOD PROFILE

- **BONES AND JOINTS** Arthritis (rheumatoid).

- **BLOOD AND CIRCULATION** Atherosclerosis, arteriosclerosis,
  high blood pressure.

- **DIGESTIVE SYSTEM** Ulcerative colitis.

- **SKIN, HAIR AND NAILS** Eczema, psoriasis.

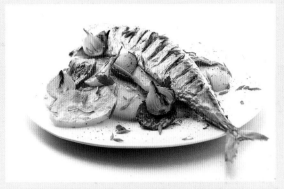

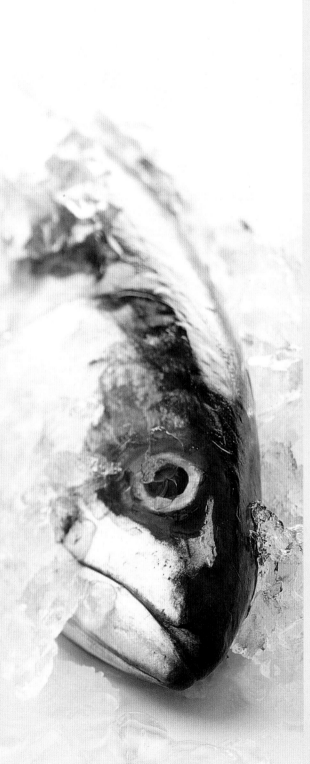

cotriade of mackerel

3 potatoes, sliced
2 medium tomatoes, sliced
150 g small onions, halved
2 cloves
2 cloves of garlic
1 bouquet garni
Pinch of saffron
Salt and pepper
150 ml dry white wine
300 ml water
1 kg mackerel, cleaned and gutted
2 tablespoons chopped parsley or chives

Spread the potatoes on the bottom of a large, well-oiled ovenproof dish. Add the other ingredients, except the parsley or chives. Put the dish in a preheated oven at 200ºC/gas mark 6 for 20 minutes or until the fish is cooked. Serve hot or warm sprinkled with parsley or chives.

honey and ginger grilled salmon

800 g salmon fillet
5 cm piece ginger root, peeled and grated
2 cloves of garlic
3 tablespoons soya sauce
½ teaspoon Chinese five spice powder
2 tablespoons clear honey
2 spring onions, chopped

In a large bowl, combine all of the ingredients. Mix well, cover with cling film and refrigerate for 30 minutes. Remove the salmon from the marinade (keep the marinade) and pat dry. Grill or pan fry for 5 minutes on either side, brushing with the marinade during cooking.

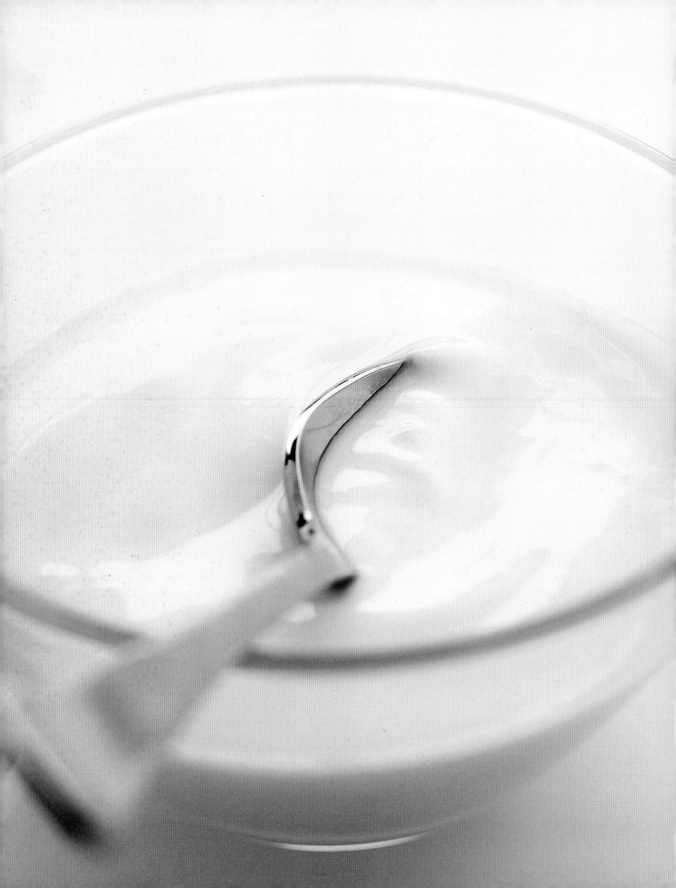

part two

foods for common ailments

When the body is fighting disease it needs all the help it can get – informed dietary choices can provide this help. To guide you through these choices, the following pages list over 100 ailments, organized by the body system that they affect. Symptom profiles, lists of beneficial foods and foods to avoid, menu suggestions to ensure the healthy function of each body system and page references to useful recipes are all designed to help you to help your body combat illness and glow with health.

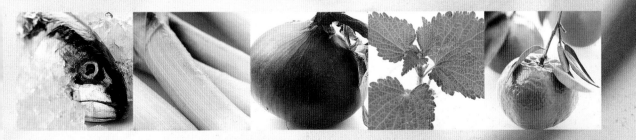

bones and joints

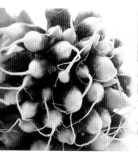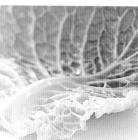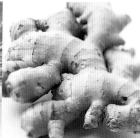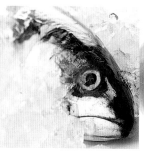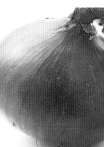

STAR FOODS FOR BONES AND JOINTS: ARTICHOKE, CABBAGE, CHEESE, CUCUMBER, DANDELION, FISH OIL, GINGER, GREEN BEAN, LEEK, MILK, NETTLE, OILY FISH, ONION, RADISH.

Our muscles, bones and joints suffer constantly from small traumas during everyday use. The musculo-skeletal system also changes gradually over the years, which may result in pain, stiffness, inflammation or some restriction of movement.

Good circulation and the elimination of uric acid are important factors in retaining maximum mobility and staying free of aches and pains. To protect your bones and joints, a constitutional approach is best: avoid alcohol, acid-forming foods and too much red meat; increase your intake of foods that are rich in minerals (such as green beans), foods that promote detoxification (artichokes, dandelion, radishes) and foods that are diuretic (cucumber, leeks, onions). Calcium and vitamin D help to strengthen the bones – calcium-rich foods include cheese, milk and fresh vegetables, and oily fish is a good source of vitamin D. Juices and infusions are useful for both bone mineralization and the elimination of waste. If you suffer from chronic arthritis or rheumatism, you should follow a strict detox programme (such as the one outlined on pages 128–31) at regular intervals.

Regular gentle exercise helps you to stay mobile. Excess weight can have an adverse effect on weight-bearing joints, such as the hips, knees and the lower part of the spine. If you experience pain or discomfort in these joints, you may need to consider losing weight by following a low-calorie diet. (N.B. To make a medicinal infusion, steep 1 tablespoon of the dried ingredient in a cup of boiling water for 10 minutes.)

ARTHRITIS (RHEUMATOID)

PAIN, INFLAMMATION AND SWELLING IN ANY OF THE JOINTS WITH OVERALL ACHING OR STIFFNESS. ARTHRITIS IS A CHRONIC, HEREDITARY ILLNESS INVOLVING AN AUTO-IMMUNE REACTION.

! ALLERGIES TO DAIRY, WHEAT, FAT OR OTHER FOOD CAN SOMETIMES EXACERBATE OR EVEN TRIGGER AN ATTACK. IF YOU SUSPECT THAT THIS IS THE CASE, ELIMINATE A FOOD FROM YOUR DIET FOR 2–3 WEEKS, RE-INTRODUCE IT GRADUALLY AND MONITOR SYMPTOMS.

✔ Apple, artichoke, asparagus, banana, blackcurrant, blueberry, cabbage, cauliflower, celery, cherry, chicory, chive and spring onion, corn, cucumber, dandelion, fennel, garlic, gooseberry, grapefruit, grape and raisin, green bean, horseradish, juniper berry, lamb's lettuce, leek, lemon, lettuce, melon, millet, nettle, oily fish, onion, parsnip, pear, pepper, pineapple, potato, prune, radish, redcurrant, salsify, tarragon, thyme, tomato, vinegar, watercress. Ginger has analgesic properties and promotes circulation – massage painful joints with a combination of ginger, rosemary and juniper-berry essential oils mixed with vegetable oil (page 50).

✘ Alcohol, coffee, cooked fat and oil, dairy products, dried beans and lentils, game and poultry, peanuts, processed food, red meat, refined oils, sorrel, sugar, tea, white flour.

RECIPES carrot, cabbage and sweet pepper juice (page 15), chickpea broth (page 86), broccoli and green bean juice (page 113), pear and apple infusion (page 118), cherry-stem decoction (page 119), cherry-stem and apple decoction (page 120), strawberry-leaf decoction (page 120), cherry-leaf wine (page 122).

ANKYLOSING SPONDYLITIS

PROGRESSIVE, CHRONIC INFLAMMATION OF THE SPINE CAUSING FLARE-UPS OF PAIN AND STIFFNESS. MOST COMMON AMONG YOUNG MEN.

✔ To relieve pain, rub some olive oil infused with bay leaves, juniper berries, camomile and rosemary flowers on the affected area of the back. Take infusions of blackcurrant leaves or strawberry root and leaves. SEE ALSO Arthritis (rheumatoid).

✘ SEE Arthritis (rheumatoid).

RECIPES strawberry leaf decoction (page 120), artichoke-leaf wine (page 122).

BURSITIS

INFLAMMATION OF A FLUID-FILLED SAC (BURSA) THAT PROTECTS A JOINT FROM FRICTION. SYMPTOMS INCLUDE PAIN, SWELLING AND RESTRICTION OF MOVEMENT IN AFFECTED JOINTS, TYPICALLY THE SHOULDER, WRIST, ELBOW, KNEE AND FINGERS.

✔ Drink pear- or blackcurrant-leaf infusion. Apply a poultice of fresh cabbage leaves to the affected joints two or three times a day to reduce inflammation. SEE ALSO general advice on the care of muscles and joints.

RECIPES pear and apple infusion (page 118).

CARPAL TUNNEL SYNDROME

COMPRESSION OF A NERVE THAT TRAVELS THROUGH THE WRIST. SYMPTOMS INCLUDE PAIN THAT SHOOTS UP THE ARM, AND NUMB, TINGLING OR BURNING SENSATIONS IN THE HAND AND FINGERS. MAY BE HORMONAL (IT CAN OCCUR SPONTANEOUSLY DURING PREGNANCY), OR CAUSED BY A REPETITIVE STRAIN INJURY.

✔ Frequent application of a poultice of cabbage leaves or a mixture of green clay, cabbage leaves (processed in a blender) and mashed cucumber may help to reduce pain and inflammation in the wrist. SEE ALSO general advice on the care of bones and joints and Bursitis.

SUGGESTED MENUS FOR INFLAMED JOINTS AND OTHER PAINFUL JOINT CONDITIONS

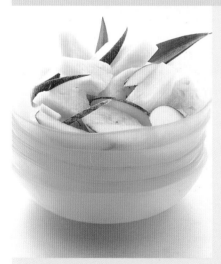

The following menus are designed for people suffering from arthritis, rheumatism, joint pain and inflammation, fibrositis or polymyalgia rheumatica, and include foods that have anti-inflammatory properties. Arthritis sufferers whose condition is exacerbated by an allergy to alcohol, dairy products or wheat should avoid the foods marked with an asterisk.

MENU 1

BREAKFAST

A bowl of sugar-free porridge with skimmed milk*, yoghurt* and a small glass of juice made from green beans, cabbage or other vegetables; or a fruit juice combination such as pineapple, apple and strawberry.

SNACKS

Dried fruit, especially raisins or apricots, and dandelion or roast-chicory coffee.

LUNCH

Chickpea or leek and potato soup with brown bread*; a mixed salad of lamb's lettuce, green beans and radishes with olive oil and lemon juice; poached salmon with potatoes; a pear or an apple.

DINNER

Steamed vegetables with ginger and garlic and a small amount of rice or noodles; an infusion of dandelion or blackcurrant leaves or a small glass of artichoke-leaf wine*.

MENU 2

BREAKFAST

A bowl of cottage cheese* mixed with two or three tablespoons of yoghurt*, a glass of fruit juice (grape, apple or cherry) and a slice of melon or a banana.

SNACKS

Dried fruit, especially blackcurrants or raisins, and dandelion or roast-chicory coffee.

LUNCH

Pasta with vegetables, smoked salmon and brown bread*; a piece of fruit.

DINNER

A mixed salad with brown bread*; an infusion of camomile or blackcurrant leaves or a small glass of artichoke-leaf wine*.

CHRONIC BACK PAIN

! MAY REQUIRE OSTEOPATHIC OR CHIROPRACTIC TREATMENT.

✔ SEE Arthritis (rheumatoid) and Osteoarthritis.

CRAMPS (MUSCULAR)

A SUDDEN MUSCULAR SPASM CAUSING TEMPORARY PAIN AND DISCOMFORT — MAY BE DUE TO A CIRCULATORY PROBLEM.

✔ Tarragon is well known for its anti-spasmodic action. Eat plenty of magnesium-rich foods, such as whole-grain cereals, nuts, seeds, seafood and green vegetables. SEE ALSO general advice in Heart and circulation.

FIBROSITIS

MUSCULAR STIFFNESS IN AREAS SUCH AS THE BACK, NECK AND SHOULDERS CAUSED BY DEPOSITS OF LACTIC AND URIC ACID AROUND THE MUSCLE FIBRES.

✔ Massage some olive oil infused with rosemary and juniper or bay berries into the affected area. SEE ALSO Arthritis (rheumatoid), Gout and Ankylosing spondylitis.

GOUT

SUDDEN ATTACK OF SEVERE PAIN, SWELLING AND INFLAMMATION, OFTEN IN THE BIG TOES, ANKLES, KNEES OR ELBOWS, OWING TO A BUILD-UP OF URIC ACID CRYSTALS IN THE JOINTS. RECURRENT ATTACKS MAY BE FREQUENT.

✔ Basil, celery, chervil, nettle, raisin, raspberry, rosemary, strawberry. Apply a poultice of fresh cabbage leaves to affected joints to reduce pain and inflammation. SEE ALSO Arthritis (rheumatoid).

✘ Tea, coffee, rhubarb.

RECIPES apple and raspberry juice (page 111), dandelion infusion (page 117), strawberry-leaf decoction (page 120), artichoke-leaf tincture (page 124).

OSTEOARTHRITIS

A CHRONIC, DEGENERATIVE CONDITION AFFECTING MOSTLY WEIGHT-BEARING JOINTS, COMMON IN THOSE AGED 40 AND OVER.

✔ Apple, asparagus, blackcurrant, cabbage, celery, chervil, bean, dandelion, ginger, leek, olive, radish, salsify, yoghurt. Drink fresh vegetable or fruit juice every day and increase the amount of oily fish, fish oil and shellfish in your diet. SEE ALSO general advice on Bones and joints.

OSTEOPOROSIS

LITERALLY "POROUS BONE" — A GRADUAL LOSS OF CALCIUM CAUSES BONES TO BECOME WEAK, BRITTLE AND PRONE TO FRACTURE. OSTEOPOROSIS IS COMMON IN POSTMENOPAUSAL WOMEN WHO HAVE LOW OESTROGEN LEVELS (THIS HORMONE REGULATES THE UPTAKE OF CALCIUM).

! A CALCIUM- AND MAGNESIUM-RICH DIET MUST BE SUPPORTED BY REGULAR LOW-INTENSITY EXERCISE AND EXPOSURE TO SUNLIGHT.

✔ Cottage cheese, fish oil, fresh fruit, goat's cheese, all green leafy vegetables, hard cheese such as Parmesan, oily fish, soya, tofu, yoghurt.

POLYMYALGIA RHEUMATICA

INFLAMMATION OF CONNECTIVE TISSUE AROUND A GROUP OF MUSCLES CAUSING PAIN, STIFFNESS AND MILD FEVER.

✔ SEE Anaemia (page 63), Arthritis (rheumatoid) and Fibrositis.

RESTLESS LEGS SYNDROME

BURNING, ACHING SENSATION IN THE LEGS CAUSING RESTLESSNESS AND TWITCHING. THE SUFFERER BECOMES IRRITABLE AND FIDGETY.

! MAY BE ASSOCIATED WITH IRON AND VITAMIN-B DEFICIENCY.

✔ Take infusions of camomile, elderberry, ginger, lemon balm, limeflower, rosemary. Use ginger, chillies and rosemary regularly in cooking. SEE ALSO general advice in Heart and Circulation.

✘ Tea, coffee.

RECIPES lemon-balm and camomile infusion (page 118), elder and camomile infusion (page 118), ginger infusion (page 119).

RHEUMATISM

ANY DISEASE THAT IS CHARACTERIZED BY INFLAMMATION IN THE MUSCLES AND JOINTS, PARTICULARLY RHEUMATOID ARTHRITIS.

✔ SEE Arthritis (rheumatoid) and Fibrositis.

TENDINITIS

INFLAMMATION OF A TENDON (THE FIBROUS TISSUE THAT CONNECTS MUSCLES AND BONES).

✔ SEE Bursitis.

TENOSYNOVITIS

INFLAMMATION OF A TENDON AND THE PROTECTIVE SHEATH THAT SURROUNDS IT.

✔ SEE Bursitis.

heart and circulation

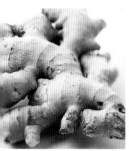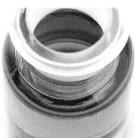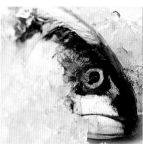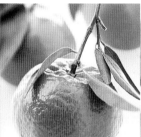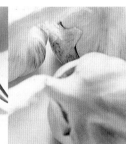

STAR FOODS FOR HEART AND CIRCULATION: BARLEY, BUCKWHEAT, CHICORY, CLOVE, GARLIC, GINGER, GREEN BEAN, LEEK, LEMON, LETTUCE, LIME, OAT, OILY FISH, OLIVE OIL, OLIVE, ONION, ORANGE, PARSLEY, PARSNIP, POTATO, PULSES, ROSEMARY, SHALLOT AND SPINACH.

Diet plays a fundamental role in the health of the heart and blood vessels. A good diet can help to keep the cardiovascular system working efficiently throughout life whereas a bad diet is a major risk factor for hypertension, atherosclerosis, heart attack and stroke. The Western diet, which tends to be high in saturated fat, sugar and salt encourages the development of fatty deposits, known as atheroma, in the arteries. The arteries narrow and problems such as blood clots and heart attacks become more likely.

If you have suffered a heart attack, the most effective way to avoid a second attack is to follow a diet that protects your cardiovascular system. Increase your intake of oily fish and fibre-rich foods; eat more potassium-rich vegetables, garlic, ginger, green vegetables and fruit, as these may help to lower your blood pressure. Bioflavonoids, found in yellow, orange, red and green vegetables and fruit, are antioxidants that help to reduce the formation of fatty deposits and clots in the arteries. Reduce your consumption of red or fatty meat (especially pork), full-fat dairy products, eggs, sugar, salt and alcohol. Eliminate fried and fast foods from your diet. Take regular, low intensity exercise, such as swimming, cycling, walking or jogging, three times a week for at least one hour at a time. If you are overweight, start following a low-calorie diet. If you smoke, it is vital that you make every effort to give up. (N.B. To make a medicinal infusion, steep 1 tablespoon of the dried ingredient in a cup of boiling water for 10 minutes.)

ANAEMIA

A DEFICIENCY OF IRON IN THE BLOOD, COMMONLY CAUSED BY A LACK OF IRON-RICH FOODS IN THE DIET OR BY A LOSS OF BLOOD, OFTEN THROUGH HEAVY MENSTRUATION. PERNICIOUS ANAEMIA IS CAUSED BY AN INABILITY TO ABSORB VITAMIN B_{12}.

✔ Iron-rich foods: apricot (dried), beetroot, blackberry, black-currant, broccoli, carrot, chervil, chestnut, dandelion, fresh fruit and vegetable juices, green bean, lamb's lettuce, nettle, parsley, prune, royal jelly, spinach, watercress. Vitamin B-rich foods: lean red meat, molasses, yeast extract. Drink plenty of fresh fruit and vegetable juices including blackberry, black cherry, grape, lettuce, spinach, fennel. If you are a vegetarian, it may be helpful to take a daily vitamin B_{12} supplement (this should be available from most health shops).

RECIPES nettle soup (page 88), cabbage, carrot and celery juice (page 113), green bean and garlic juice (page 113), broccoli and green bean juice (page 113), celery and red onion juice (page 113), fennel infusion (page 117), fennel-seed decoction (page 120), blackcurrant wine (page 121).

ANGINA

TEMPORARY SENSATIONS OF PRESSURE OR PAIN IN THE CENTRE OF THE CHEST RESULTING FROM POOR BLOOD SUPPLY TO THE HEART. USUALLY CAUSED BY BLOCKED AND NARROWED ARTERIES. ATTACKS ARE TRIGGERED BY STRESS AND EXERTION.

! DO NOT STOP TAKING MEDICATION PRESCRIBED BY YOUR DOCTOR.

SEVERE CHEST PAIN THAT IS NOT ALLEVIATED BY REST SHOULD BE
TREATED AS A MEDICAL EMERGENCY.

✔ Eat a small portion of oily fish every day. Increase your intake of
magnesium-rich food, such as whole-grain cereal products, nuts
and seeds. Drink infusions of olive leaves and limeflower. *SEE ALSO*
Atherosclerosis, Arteriosclerosis, High blood pressure and Stress-
related symptoms (page 77).

✘ Fatty red meat, full-fat dairy products (such as butter, high-fat
cheese and double cream), egg, sugary foods, salt and alcohol.
Avoid fried and fast foods.

*RECIPES garlic tincture (page 48), green bean and garlic juice
(page 113), broccoli and green bean juice (page 113), celery and
red onion juice (page 113), lemon-balm and camomile infusion
(page 118), ginger infusion (page 119).*

ATHEROSCLEROSIS

THE CLOGGING UP OF ARTERIES BY FATTY DEPOSITS KNOWN AS
ATHEROMAS. THIS CONDITION IS DIRECTLY LINKED TO AN EXCESS OF
FAT AND SUGAR IN THE DIET.

❗ DO NOT STOP TAKING MEDICATION PRESCRIBED BY YOUR DOCTOR.

✔ Apricot, blackcurrant, blueberry, celery, cherry, fig, garlic,
germinated barley, ginger, grape, lemon, oat, olive, pineapple,
prune, sage, seaweed. Eat oily fish as often as possible and plenty
of yellow, orange, red and green, leafy vegetables. Take artichoke,
blackcurrant (leaves and fruit) and strawberry-leaf infusions or
decoctions. Drink blueberry juice.

✘ Fatty red meat, full-fat dairy products, fried or oily foods, fast
and processed foods, foods that are high in sugar.

*RECIPES cabbage, carrot and blueberry juice (page 19), cabbage,
carrot and celery juice (page 113), ginger infusion (page 119),
strawberry-leaf decoction (page 120), barley water (page 121).*

ARTERIOSCLEROSIS

THE HARDENING OF ARTERIES IN OLD AGE, A CONDITION OFTEN
ACCELERATED OR AGGRAVATED BY A DIET THAT CONTAINS AN EXCESS
OF ALCOHOL, FAT, SALT AND SUGAR.

❗ DO NOT STOP TAKING MEDICATION PRESCRIBED BY YOUR DOCTOR.

✔ Apricot, artichoke leaf, asparagus, black radish, blueberry,
camomile, celery, chicory, dandelion, fish, garlic, grape, lamb's
lettuce, lettuce, limeflower, onion, orange, parsley, pineapple,
potato, pumpkin, raspberry, rosemary, rye, saffron, spring onion
and chive, strawberry. *SEE ALSO* Atherosclerosis.

✘ Alcohol, fast and processed foods, fatty red meat, fried or oily
foods, full-fat dairy products, salt, sugar.

*RECIPES garlic tincture (page 48), strawberry-leaf decoction
(page 120), artichoke-leaf wine (page 122).*

SUGGESTED MENUS FOR HIGH BLOOD PRESSURE

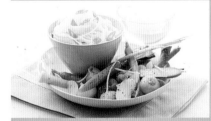

The following menus are designed to promote
weight loss and should ease symptoms
associated with stress and high blood pressure,
such as digestive problems and water retention.
The menus are also recommended for anyone
with a heart or circulatory condition. If you are
not trying to lose weight, simply increase the
amount of food in each meal.

MENU 1

BREAKFAST

A bowl of sugar-free cereal with skimmed
milk; yoghurt; a small glass of lettuce,
cucumber and garlic juice or pineapple,
apple and strawberry juice.

SNACKS

Any dried fruit; dandelion coffee substitute.

LUNCH

Lentil soup with brown bread; a salad of
fennel, radicchio and olives with olive oil
and lemon juice dressing; fish with
potatoes; a piece of fruit.

DINNER

Steamed vegetables with ginger and garlic
on a small bed of noodles (left); a small
glass of artichoke-leaf wine (page 122).

MENU 2

BREAKFAST

A bowl of porridge; grape or apple juice.

SNACKS

Any dried fruit; dandelion coffee substitute.

LUNCH

Leek and potato soup; cottage cheese,
smoked salmon and brown bread; a piece
of fruit.

DINNER

A mixed salad with brown bread; an
infusion of camomile or blackcurrant leaves.

CHILBLAINS

PAINFUL, ITCHY SWELLINGS OF THE SKIN CAUSED BY EXPOSURE TO COLD AND POOR CIRCULATION.

✔ To improve circulation: blackcurrant, blackberry, blueberry, cabbage, carrot, chervil, garlic, ginger, redcurrant. Consume a lot of warm food and drinks. Drink blackberry-leaf infusion. *SEE ALSO* Anaemia.

RECIPES ginger infusion (page 119).

HIGH BLOOD PRESSURE

HIGH BLOOD PRESSURE (HYPERTENSION) OCCURS WHEN THERE IS RESISTANCE IN THE BLOOD VESSELS TO THE FLOW OF BLOOD. IT IS OFTEN SYMPTOMLESS OR ASSOCIATED WITH HIGH CHOLESTEROL AND ARTERIOSCLEROSIS. RISK FACTORS INCLUDE CHRONIC STRESS, AGE, POOR DIET AND EXCESSIVE ALCOHOL CONSUMPTION. HIGH BLOOD PRESSURE GREATLY INCREASES THE PATIENT'S RISK OF SUFFERING A STROKE OR HEART ATTACK.

! DO NOT STOP TAKING MEDICATION PRESCRIBED BY YOUR DOCTOR.

✔ Artichoke, asparagus, broccoli, celery, dandelion, garlic, grape, leek, lettuce, oat, oily fish, olive and olive oil, olive-leaf infusion, onion, pomegranate, potassium-rich vegetables, red wine, rice, rye, sunflower seeds and oil, tomato. Increase your intake of magnesium-rich food, such as whole-grain cereal products, nuts and seeds. In many cases, overcoming obesity is the most effective way of lowering high blood pressure – follow a low-calorie, dairy-free, wheat-free diet for as long as necessary. Combine this diet with regular low-intensity, prolonged exercise. Drink grape juice and infusions of artichoke and olive leaf. *SEE ALSO* Atherosclerosis.

✘ High-fat foods, including dairy products, and wheat.

RECIPES cabbage, carrot and blueberry juice (page 19), garlic tincture (page 48), celery and tomato juice (page 112), green bean and garlic juice (page 113), celery and red onion juice (page 113), cucumber and lettuce heart juice (page 113), lettuce and basil juice (page 113), dandelion infusion (page 117).

HYPERLIPIDAEMIA

AN EXCESSIVE AMOUNT OF FAT IN THE BLOOD. OFTEN LINKED TO HEAVY ALCOHOL CONSUMPTION, SMOKING, LACK OF EXERCISE AND A DIET THAT IS HIGH IN FAT.

! DO NOT STOP TAKING MEDICATION PRESCRIBED BY YOUR DOCTOR.

✔ Celeriac, dandelion, fig, garlic, germinated barley, nuts, oat, oily fish, onion, papaya. Drink infusions of artichoke and olive leaf.

Include plenty of olive oil in your diet. *SEE ALSO* Atherosclerosis and Arteriosclerosis.

✘ Avoid fatty foods, except oily fish.

RECIPES garlic tincture (page 48), artichoke-leaf wine (page 122).

PALPITATIONS/ARRHYTHMIA

AN IRREGULAR HEARTBEAT, WHICH MAY BE CAUSED BY CONGENITAL FACTORS, OR MAY BE THE RESULT OF EXERTION, STRESS OR HEART DISEASE.

! DO NOT STOP TAKING MEDICATION PRESCRIBED BY YOUR DOCTOR.

✔ Buckwheat, chicory, clove, garlic, germinated barley, green bean, leek, lemon, lemon balm, lettuce, limeflower, mint, parsley, parsnip, passion fruit, oat, olive leaf (in infusion) and oil, onion, rosemary, shallot, tarragon, valerian.

✘ Alcohol, coffee, tea, tobacco.

RECIPES green bean and garlic juice (page 113), celery and red onion juice (page 113), lettuce and basil juice (page 113), lemon-balm and camomile infusion (page 118), barley water (page 121).

THROMBOSIS

FORMATION OF A BLOOD CLOT WITHIN A BLOOD VESSEL OR INSIDE THE HEART, OFTEN IMPEDING THE FLOW OF BLOOD.

! DO NOT STOP TAKING MEDICATION PRESCRIBED BY YOUR DOCTOR.

✔ Borage oil, buckwheat, camomile, fenugreek, garlic, lemon, limeflower, oily fish, olive oil, orange, pineapple, pumpkin, raspberry, strawberry, tarragon. Eat oily fish on a regular basis.

✘ Alcohol, tobacco.

RECIPES garlic tincture (page 48), strawberry and raspberry juice (page 112), green bean and garlic juice (page 113), celery and red onion juice (page 113), strawberry-leaf decoction (page 120).

RAYNAUD'S DISEASE

INADEQUATE CIRCULATION IN THE HANDS OR FEET DUE TO ARTERIAL SPASM CAUSES FINGERS OR TOES TO TURN WHITE OR BLUE AND STING ON EXPOSURE TO COLD. THE CHEEKS, EARS AND NOSE MAY ALSO BE AFFECTED.

✔ Blackberry, blackcurrant, black pepper, blueberry, cabbage, carrot, cayenne pepper, chervil, cinnamon, garlic, ginger, red-currant. Consume a lot of warm food and drinks. Raise your intake of magnesium-rich food, such as whole-grain cereal products, nuts and seeds. Drink blackberry leaf infusion. *SEE ALSO* Anaemia.

RECIPES ginger infusion (page 119).

digestive system

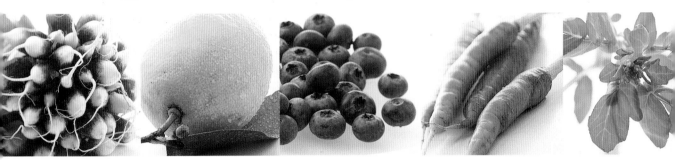

STAR FOODS FOR THE DIGESTIVE SYSTEM: ALL BITTER GREENS, ARTICHOKE, BASIL, BLACKCURRANT, BLACK RADISH, BLUEBERRY, CARROT, CHERVIL, CHICORY, COURGETTE, DANDELION, FENNEL, FIG, GARLIC, GERMINATED BARLEY, GINGER, GRAPEFRUIT, JUNIPER BERRY, LEMON, LETTUCE, OLIVE OIL, PAPAYA, PARSLEY, PINEAPPLE, NUTMEG, QUINCE, RADISH, ROSEMARY, THYME, WATERCRESS.

The digestive system includes the mouth, oesophagus, stomach, liver, pancreas, gallbladder and intestines. A diet that consists largely of convenience foods and is high in sugar and fat – as well as alcohol, fizzy drinks, spicy snacks and tobacco – puts the digestive tract under constant strain. The digestive system is also notoriously sensitive to stress and emotional conditions. If you often experience minor digestive problems, or suffer from a chronic condition, you should try to reduce your stress levels as much as possible.

Many digestive problems can be alleviated by eliminating alcohol, coffee, spicy or salty snacks, fatty food (such as cream, cheese and butter) and junk food from your diet. Eating less, but at regular intervals, can also help. Increase your food intake in the morning, eat moderately at lunchtime and lightly in the evening. Some people feel better if they eat five small meals a day.

Two or three times a year, go on a wheat- and dairy-free diet for two to three weeks at a time, or follow the detox program outlined on pages 128–31. Fibre encourages food to pass quickly though the gut so try to increase the amount you include in your diet by eating plenty of fresh vegetables (don't just rely on cereals as a source of fibre). When cooking, use plenty of herbs, such as basil, garlic, ginger, juniper, rosemary and thyme – these are naturally antibacterial and promote digestion. Cabbage, carrots, courgettes, lettuce, fennel,

blueberries, figs, papaya and pineapple are beneficial to both the stomach and the intestines; germinated barley is good for dyspepsia. Efficient liver function is important for healthy digestion – bitter greens, artichokes, blackcurrant berries and leaves, black radishes, chervil, chicory, dandelion, grapefruit, lemon, olive oil, parsley, quince and watercress all help the liver to function efficiently. They also promote the flow and emulsification of bile. (N.B. To make a medicinal infusion, steep 1 tablespoon of the dried ingredient in a cup of boiling water for 10 minutes.)

ABDOMINAL PAIN

SUDDEN ACUTE ABDOMINAL PAIN, WHICH MAY BE ACCOMPANIED BY SWELLING OF THE ABDOMEN, DIARRHOEA OR VOMITING.

! MAY RAPIDLY TURN INTO A MEDICAL EMERGENCY – SEE A DOCTOR AS SOON AS POSSIBLE. USE SELF-HELP MEASURES ONLY WHEN POTENTIALLY SERIOUS CONDITIONS HAVE BEEN RULED OUT.

ABDOMINAL CRAMP

DISCOMFORT IN THE ABDOMEN MAY BE DUE TO TRAPPED WIND, CONSTIPATION OR IRRITABLE BOWEL SYNDROME.

✔ Infusions of aniseed, basil, bay leaf, camomile, coriander, cumin seed, dill, fennel seed, ginger, lemon balm, lychee seed, marjoram, mint, oregano, tarragon. Blueberry, cucumber, carrot and garlic may alleviate intestinal fermentation and inflammation. SEE ALSO general advice on the digestive system and Distention and wind.

RECIPES cabbage, carrot and blueberry juice (page 19), blueberry decoction (page 34), cucumber and lettuce heart juice (page 113), fennel infusion (page 117), lemon-balm and camomile infusion (page 118), lychee-seed decoction (page 120), dill-seed decoction (page 120), fennel-seed decoction (page 120), cumin-seed decoction (page 120), camomile and citrus wine (page 123), anisette (page 123), basil liqueur (page 123).

BLOATING

SEE ABDOMINAL PAIN, DISTENTION AND WIND.

CHOLECYSTITIS

AN ACUTE OR CHRONIC INFLAMMATION OF THE GALLBLADDER, OWING TO A BLOCKAGE (USUALLY BY GALLSTONES) OR AN INFECTION, CAUSING PAIN IN THE UPPER RIGHT ABDOMEN AND/OR BETWEEN THE SHOULDERS. THE CONDITION IS OFTEN ACCOMPANIED BY INDIGESTION AND NAUSEA AFTER EATING FATTY FOOD.

! ACUTE PAIN MAY RAPIDLY TURN INTO A MEDICAL EMERGENCY – SEE A DOCTOR AS SOON AS POSSIBLE. USE SELF-HELP MEASURES ONLY WHEN POTENTIALLY SERIOUS CONDITIONS HAVE BEEN RULED OUT.

✔ Bitter greens, dandelion, fresh fruit and vegetables, hazelnut. Try to use plenty of rosemary in your cooking. Every morning drink some olive oil mixed with lemon juice (see page 28) followed by a glass of black radish and carrot juice (see below). Artichoke-leaf, lemon, lemon-peel or rosemary infusions or fresh cherry juice may also provide some relief.

✘ Biscuits and other refined carbohydrates, fatty foods, rhubarb.

RECIPES cherry and raspberry juice (page 112), cherry and apple juice (page 112), black radish and carrot juice (page 113), dandelion infusion (page 117), artichoke-leaf wine (page 122), lemon liqueur (page 123), artichoke-leaf tincture (page 124).

COLIC

SEE ABDOMINAL CRAMP, CONSTIPATION, INDIGESTION.

SUGGESTED MENUS TO AID DIGESTION

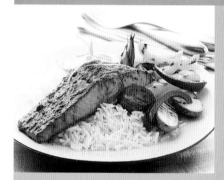

The following menus are helpful for anyone suffering from minor problems, such as constipation, distention and wind, that are caused by a weak or sluggish digestive system.

MENU 1

BREAKFAST

A bowl of porridge; yoghurt; a small glass of juice made of carrot, cabbage and green or red pepper; or a fruit juice combination such as blackcurrant, blueberry and blackberry or pineapple, apple and strawberry.

SNACKS

Dried fruit, especially blueberries, pineapple or papaya; dandelion or roast-chicory coffee substitute; fennel, ginger and basil infusion or lemon-balm infusion.

LUNCH

Fish or chicken with potatoes and herb sauce (page 105) or buckwheat with leek sauce (page 97) or taboule (page 94) with a grilled lamb chop and a carrot and orange salad; rhubarb and ginger tart (page 107).

DINNER

Broad-bean soup or herbal broth (page 86) cooked with barley; fresh fruit salad; a camomile infusion; a small glass of basil liqueur (page 123) or a teaspoon of anisette (page 123) in a glass of water.

MENU 2

BREAKFAST

A bowl of rice or corn flakes with soya milk or an autumn fruit compote; fruit juice (grape, apple or blueberry); half a grapefruit, a banana or a kiwi fruit.

SNACKS

Dried fruit, especially raisins, papaya, pineapple or blueberries; dandelion or roast-chicory coffee substitute; fennel, ginger or cumin-seed infusion.

LUNCH

Honey and ginger grilled salmon (page 57) with steamed vegetables; pumpkin in syrup (page 106).

DINNER

Roman-style artichoke (page 95) or red lentil soup (page 89); pears with herbs (page 108); a small glass of camomile and citrus wine (page 123).

COLITIS

SEE ABDOMINAL PAIN, IRRITABLE BOWEL SYNDROME, ULCERATIVE COLITIS.

CONSTIPATION

SLOW INTESTINAL TRANSIT CAUSING IRREGULAR BOWEL MOVEMENTS.

! STRONG LAXATIVES SHOULD BE AVOIDED. A HIGH-FIBRE DIET AND AN INCREASED INTAKE OF RAW FRUIT AND VEGETABLES OFTEN HELPS TO RELIEVE THIS CONDITION.

✔ All green leafy vegetables, apple, asparagus, Brussels sprout, chervil, coconut, cooked rhubarb, cucumber, elderberry, fig, grapefruit, hazelnut, Jerusalem artichoke, kumquat, leek, live yoghurt, melon, mustard, olive, orange, peach, pea, persimmon, pomegranate, prune, raspberry, raw apple, redcurrant, sorrel, strawberry, turnip, tomato, watermelon. Drink plenty of water and fresh apple, melon, prune or tomato juice – mix the juice with yoghurt if desired. Every morning drink some olive oil mixed with lemon juice (page 28) and eat some figs boiled in milk (page 30).

✘ Guava seeds. If the condition worsens when you eat foods that contain wheat, you should suspect a wheat allergy and eliminate it from your diet.

RECIPES almond milk (page 71), rhubarb and ginger tart (page 107), apple and raspberry juice (page 111), prune juice (page 112), celery and tomato juice (page 112), cucumber and lettuce heart juice (page 113), elderberry syrup (page 125).

CROHN'S DISEASE

A RECURRENT INFLAMMATION OF THE INTESTINE WHICH MAY NECESSITATE SURGERY. SYMPTOMS – WHICH ARE NOT ALWAYS PRESENT, EVEN IN SERIOUS CASES – INCLUDE CRAMPING PAIN, DIARRHOEA, WEIGHT LOSS, ANAEMIA AND SOMETIMES JOINT PAIN.

! DO NOT STOP TAKING MEDICATION PRESCRIBED BY YOUR DOCTOR.

✔ Almond, blueberry, cabbage, carrot, courgette, fig, ginger, grapefruit, mint, peach, pumpkin, pollen, quince, tarragon. Aniseed or mint infusion or fennel tea may also provide some relief. SEE ALSO general advice on the care of the digestive system.

✘ Guava seeds and all dairy products except live yoghurt.

RECIPES cabbage, carrot and blueberry juice (page 19), almond milk (page 71), cabbage, carrot and celery juice (page 113), fennel infusion (page 117), coriander-seed infusion (page 119), anisette (page 123), quince liqueur (page 123).

DIABETES MELLITUS

A CHRONIC CONDITION IN WHICH AN ABSENCE OR INSUFFICIENCY OF INSULIN LEADS TO PROBLEMS IN THE METABOLISM OF SUGAR. AS A RESULT, SUGAR BUILDS UP IN THE BLOOD AND URINE.

! DO NOT STOP TAKING MEDICATION PRESCRIBED BY YOUR DOCTOR. YOUR DOCTOR MAY REFER YOU TO A REGISTERED DIETICIAN.

✔ Artichoke, bean, blueberry, brown bread and pasta, brown flour, cabbage, chive and spring onion, fresh fruit, garlic, Jerusalem artichoke, nut, oat, olive, onion, potato, pulses, pumpkin, salsify, shallot, rice, unrefined cereals. Drink fresh blueberry, cabbage, celery or citrus-fruit juice and blueberry, blueberry-leaf or juniper infusion.

✘ Excessive amounts of animal fat. Consult your doctor before eating bananas.

RECIPES blueberry tincture (page 34), cabbage, carrot and celery juice (page 113), beetroot and celery juice (page 113), juniper-berry wine (page 122).

DIARRHOEA

THE PASSING OF FREQUENT LIQUID STOOLS CAUSED BY PARASITES, BACTERIAL OR VIRAL ACTIVITY, FOOD INTOLERANCE, STRESS OR DRUGS.

! DIARRHOEA CAN CAUSE RAPID DEHYDRATION. SEE YOUR DOCTOR IF THE ATTACK IS PROLONGED.

✔ Barley, blackberry, blueberry, boiled carrot, boiled rice, broad bean, cabbage, camomile, cardamom, chilli, chive, clove, cooked apple, honey, lychee, nettle, nutmeg, onion, pear, peppercorns, pepper, quince, rice water, rosemary, savory, strawberry, walnut. Drink fresh blackberry, blueberry or carrot juice and fennel-seed or rice-water infusion.

RECIPES blueberry decoction (page 34), blueberry tincture (page 34), fennel infusion (page 117), fennel-seed decoction (page 120), quince liqueur (page 123), blackberry syrup (page 125).

DISTENTION AND WIND

ABDOMINAL BLOATING, DISCOMFORT OR PAIN CAUSED BY FERMENTATION OF FOOD, EXCESS YEAST, BACTERIAL ACTIVITY OR STRESS.

✔ Anise, blackberry, blueberry, carrot, chilli, garlic, lettuce, marjoram, oregano, pepper, savory. Use plenty of bay leaf, clove, coriander, cumin seed, fennel, juniper and rosemary in your cooking. Drink fresh blackberry, blueberry or lettuce and garlic juice and aniseed, camomile, cumin-seed, dill-seed or fennel-seed infusion.

✘ Alcohol, fermented foods and foods that may ferment, such as bread, flour-based foods, pulses and sugary foods.
RECIPES bay-leaf infusion (page 44), lettuce and basil juice (page 113), dill-seed decoction (page 120), fennel-seed decoction (page 120), cumin-seed decoction (page 120).

DIVERTICULITIS

SMALL POUCHES IN THE LARGE INTESTINE WHICH BECOME INFLAMED, CAUSING PAIN, WIND, DIARRHOEA OR CONSTIPATION.

✔ High-fibre foods: apple, bean, blackberry, blueberry, brown bread, brown rice, Brussels sprout, cabbage, chestnut, chickpea, dried fruit, grapefruit, green vegetables, Jerusalem artichoke, lentil, melon, orange, parsnip, pea, porridge, potato, turnip, watermelon. As some of these foods may increase the production of gas, use plenty of fresh herbs and garlic in your cooking.

✘ Guava seeds.
RECIPES cabbage, carrot and blueberry juice (page 19), garlic and sage soup (page 49), cucumber and lettuce heart juice (page 113), fennel infusion (page 117), lemon-balm and camomile infusion (page 118), dill-seed decoction (page 120), fennel-seed decoction (page 120), cumin-seed decoction (page 120), anisette (page 123).

DYSENTERY

SEE ABDOMINAL PAIN, DIARRHOEA.

✘ Pumpkin.

DYSPEPSIA AND HEARTBURN

INDIGESTION AND A BURNING SENSATION IN THE CHEST, OFTEN DUE TO RICH OR SWEET FOOD, OVEREATING, ALCOHOL OR STRESS.

✔ Anise, apple, banana, barley, bay leaf, carrot, chestnut, chilli, coriander, courgette, fennel, fig, grapefruit, guava (seeded), Jerusalem artichoke, lemon, lettuce, melon, orange, peach, peanut, peppercorns, pepper, persimmon, pineapple, potato, pumpkin, quince, radish, rocket, saffron.

✘ Alcohol, coffee, fatty food, tea. Do not eat late at night.
RECIPES lemon-balm and camomile infusion (page 118), coriander-seed infusion (page 119), fennel-seed decoction (page 120), anisette (page 123), aniseed tincture (page 124).

FLATULENCE

SEE DISTENTION AND WIND.

FOOD POISONING

SEE GASTROENTERITIS, INDIGESTION, NAUSEA AND VOMITING.

GALLSTONES

SEE CHOLECYSTITIS.

GASTRITIS

A GENERAL INFLAMMATION OF THE LINING OF THE STOMACH, CAUSING SYMPTOMS SIMILAR TO THOSE OF INDIGESTION.

✔ A 20-hour fast, drinking only barley water or rice water (see Rice; page 27) may reduce the symptoms considerably. Follow this with a diet of bland foods such as: banana, barley, cabbage, carrot, courgette, fennel, fig, Jerusalem artichoke, potato, pumpkin, quince, rice, watermelon. Drink fresh carrot, cabbage or courgette juice, and aniseed, dill-seed, fennel-seed or mint infusions. *SEE ALSO* general advice on the care of the digestive system, Dyspepsia and Indigestion.

BARLEY AND FRUIT PORRIDGE

This recipe by Hanne Glasse, which was first published in 1747, can help to boost a sluggish digestive system.

50 g germinated barley
1 litre water (or equal parts of water and milk)
25 g raisins
25 g dried blackcurrants or blueberries
Pinch of ground nutmeg
2 tablespoons brown sugar
50ml white wine or a little brandy
2 egg yolks (optional)

In a large saucepan, boil the barley in the water with the raisins, blackcurrants or blueberries and nutmeg until the barley is tender. Remove from the heat and stir in the brown sugar and white wine. Return to the heat, bring to the boil and cook over a low heat for a further 2 minutes. Add the egg yolks at this stage if desired, but remove from the heat before stirring them in. The end result should resemble rice pudding.

RECIPES cabbage, carrot and celery juice (page 113), lettuce and basil juice (page 113), coriander-seed infusion (page 119), dill-seed decoction (page 120), fennel-seed decoction (page 120).

GASTROENTERITIS

AN INFLAMMATION OF THE DIGESTIVE TRACT CAUSED BY MICRO-ORGANISMS AND RESULTING IN NAUSEA, VOMITING, DIARRHOEA, ABDOMINAL PAIN AND FEVER.

! DO NOT EAT ANYTHING FOR 24 HOURS. DRINK SMALL AMOUNTS OF FLUIDS FREQUENTLY. GINGER, FENNEL OR MINT TEA OR AN INFUSION OF THYME, JUNIPER OR BASIL MAY HELP.

✔ When you feel you can start eating again, eat very lightly, preferably food cooked with garlic and basil, juniper, marjoram, mint, rosemary or thyme to reduce the infection. Also eat: blueberry, boiled carrot, chickpea, chive and spring onion, courgette, lamb's lettuce, pumpkin, quince, persimmon, watercress.

RECIPES garlic and sage soup (page 49), almond milk (see opposite page), herbal broth (page 86), ginger infusion (page 119), fennel-seed decoction (page 120), barley water (page 121), basil liqueur (page 123).

GINGIVITIS

INFECTED OR BLEEDING GUMS, OFTEN CAUSED BY BACTERIAL ACTIVITY AND OCCASIONALLY BY VITAMIN DEFICIENCY.

! ALWAYS BRUSH TEETH AND GUMS THOROUGHLY.

✔ Chew lemon peel, cloves, fresh or dried blueberries or figs. Add a tablespoon of salt and a drop or two of lemon essential oil to a strong thyme infusion to make a mouth wash. A strong sage infusion with a teaspoon of lemon juice added also makes a good mouth wash, as does fig water (see Fig; page 30).

✘ sugary food.

HALITOSIS (BAD BREATH)

BAD BREATH IS OFTEN CAUSED BY YEAST OR BACTERIAL ACTIVITY IN THE MOUTH OF BY VARIOUS DIGESTIVE PROBLEMS.

✔ Nutmeg and an infusion of cardamom seeds. *SEE ALSO* Gingivitis.

HANGOVER

DELAYED EFFECTS OF DRINKING AN EXCESSIVE AMOUNT OF ALCOHOL, INCLUDING FATIGUE, HEADACHE, NAUSEA, INDIGESTION.

✔ Drink plenty of water and infusions throughout the day. *SEE ALSO* Indigestion.

RECIPES garlic and sage soup (page 49), dandelion infusion (page 117), fennel infusion (page 117), ginger infusion (page 119).

HEPATITIS (A, B OR C)

CHRONIC OR ACUTE INFECTION OF THE LIVER CAUSED BY A VIRUS. SYMPTOMS INCLUDE FATIGUE, INDIGESTION, JAUNDICE AND LOSS OF APPETITE.

! IT IS IMPERATIVE TO FOLLOW MEDICAL ADVICE.

✔ Bitter greens, apple, artichoke, asparagus, black radish, blueberry, cabbage, celery, chard, chervil, chicory, dandelion, grapefruit, green bean, horseradish, lemon, olive and olive oil, parsley. Drink fresh lettuce juice, mint tea or some olive oil mixed with lemon juice (page 28) .

✘ Alcohol, fatty food, meat, tobacco.

RECIPES dandelion infusion (page 117)).

INDIGESTION

A VARIETY OF SYMPTOMS, WHICH MAY INCLUDE NAUSEA, VOMITING, HEARTBURN AND BELCHING. INDIGESTION IS OFTEN CAUSED BY EXCESSIVE CONSUMPTION OF FATTY FOOD OR ALCOHOL.

✔ Drink water or take a decoction, infusion or tincture (see below). Eat as little as possible until symptoms have cleared.

RECIPES garlic and sage soup (page 49), herbal broth (page 86), fennel infusion (page 117), lemon-balm and camomile infusion (page 118), coriander-seed infusion (page 119), ginger infusion (page 119), fennel-seed decoction (page 120), aniseed tincture (page 124).

INTESTINAL INFECTIONS AND PARASITES

SEE GASTROENTERITIS

IRRITABLE BOWEL SYNDROME

ABDOMINAL CRAMPS AND SPASMS, AND ALTERNATING OR IRREGULAR BOUTS OF CONSTIPATION AND DIARRHOEA. OFTEN ASSOCIATED WITH STRESS, PSYCHOLOGICAL PROBLEMS AND CHANGE OF ROUTINE.

! AVOID ALL DAIRY PRODUCTS AND WHEAT FOR 2 WEEKS. A WEEK OR TWO LATER REINTRODUCE WHEAT, THEN DAIRY INTO YOUR DIET — IF EITHER CAUSES A SUDDEN RETURN OR AGGRAVATION OF THE CONDITION, ELIMINATE IT FROM YOUR DIET FOR GOOD.

✔ Almond milk, barley, blueberry, camomile, carrot, coriander, courgette, germinated pulses, ginger, melon, mint, persimmon, potato, quince, pumpkin, rice, rosemary, tarragon. Drink parsley-seed or mint infusion.

✗ Dairy products and wheat (if they exacerbate symptoms).
RECIPES *almond milk (see below), fennel infusion (page 117), dill-seed decoction (page 120), fennel-seed decoction (page 120), anisette (page 123), basil liqueur (page 123).*

NAUSEA AND VOMITING

MAY BE A SYMPTOM OF INDIGESTION OR GASTROENTERITIS, BUT OCCASIONALLY INDICATES A SERIOUS DISORDER.

! SEE A DOCTOR IF SYMPTOMS ARE PROLONGED. SEE A DOCTOR IMMEDIATELY IF YOU ARE IN PAIN, WORRIED ABOUT THE CAUSE OF VOMITING, OR IF THERE IS BLOOD IN THE VOMIT.

✔ Infusions of anise, fennel, ginger, mint. SEE ALSO Cholecystitis, Gastritis, Hangover, Indigestion and Migraine (page 76).
RECIPES *ginger infusion (page 119), fennel-seed decoction (page 120), basil liqueur (page 123).*

OBESITY

EXCESSIVE BODY WEIGHT WHICH IMPAIRS MOVEMENT AND MAY LEAD TO SERIOUS HEALTH DISORDERS. OBESITY IS OFTEN DUE TO HABITUAL OVEREATING COMBINED WITH A LACK OF EXERCISE. OTHER CAUSES MAY BE A SLOW METABOLISM OR A MALFUNCTIONING THYROID GLAND.

ALMOND MILK

Almond milk is helpful for people suffering from constipation, Crohn's disease, gastroenteritis, irritable bowel syndrome and ulcerative colitis. It also acts as a mild laxative for children and is also good for bronchial inflammation and coughs (page 72).

100 g almonds

1 tablespoon water

50 g clear honey

1 litre water

2 tablespoons orange-blossom water

Blend the almonds and the tablespoon of water in a food processor until you have a paste. Add the honey and then dilute the paste with the litre of water. Filter and add the orange-blossom water. Take 3 tablespoons 3 times a day.

! IT IS NOT POSSIBLE TO REDUCE WEIGHT WITHOUT DECREASING CALORIE INTAKE (EATING LESS) AND INCREASING THE RATE AT WHICH CALORIES ARE USED (EXERCISING MORE).

✔ Eat plenty of foods that are both low-calorie and high-volume, such as green vegetables, potato and pulses.

✗ Dairy products, wheat (if they cause an allergy). SEE ALSO the detox programme (pages 128–31).

PEPTIC ULCERS

INCLUDES GASTRIC AND DUODENAL ULCERS; A SMALL AREA OF THE LINING OF THE STOMACH OR DUODENUM BECOMES INFLAMED, THEN ERODED. SYMPTOMS OF PEPTIC ULCERS INCLUDE A BURNING, GNAWING PAIN IN THE UPPER ABDOMEN OR CHEST, INDIGESTION, NAUSEA AND VOMITING.

! DO NOT STOP TAKING MEDICATION PRESCRIBED BY YOUR DOCTOR. SEVERE PAIN AND VOMITING BRIGHT RED BLOOD INDICATE THAT THE ULCER HAS BECOME PERFORATED – SEE A DOCTOR IMMEDIATELY. GIVE UP SMOKING.

✔ Apple, banana, cabbage, carrot, fennel, fig, lettuce, potato, quince, rice barley. Eat small meals. Drink a potato-juice remedy (page 12) mixed with fresh carrot juice.

✗ Acidic, fatty or spicy foods, alcohol, coffee, tea.
RECIPES *cabbage, carrot and blueberry juice (page 19), fennel infusion (page 117), coriander-seed infusion (page 119), fennel-seed decoction (page 120), aniseed tincture (page 124).*

ULCERATIVE COLITIS

CHRONIC INFLAMMATION AND ULCERATION OF THE LOWER PART OF THE COLON CAUSING ABDOMINAL PAIN, AND DIARRHOEA WITH BLOOD AND MUCUS.

! DO NOT STOP TAKING MEDICATION PRESCRIBED BY YOUR DOCTOR.

✔ Barley, beetroot, blackberry, blueberry, broad bean, cabbage, carrot, cauliflower, cereals, cooked apple, courgette, cucumber, dandelion, fresh fruit and vegetables, garlic, gooseberry, lamb's lettuce, lettuce, lychee, mango, nettle, oily fish, pear, persimmon, potato, quince, rosemary, strawberry. Eat high-fibre foods and reduce your meat intake. SEE ALSO Anaemia (page 63).

✗ Alcohol, dairy products, guava seeds, tobacco.
RECIPES *almond milk (left), cabbage, carrot and blueberry juice (page 19), mango juice (page 112), fennel infusion (page 117), lemon-balm and camomile infusion (page 118), elder and camomile infusion (page 118), fennel-seed decoction (page 120).*

respiratory system

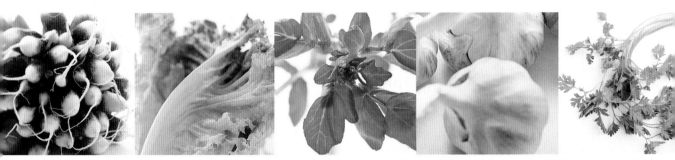

STAR FOODS FOR THE RESPIRATORY SYSTEM: BASIL, CHERVIL, CHIVE AND SPRING ONION, GARLIC, GINGER, LAMB'S LETTUCE, LETTUCE, MARJORAM, MINT, PARSLEY, RED AND BLACK RADISH, ROSEMARY, SAVORY, THYME, WATERCRESS.

Common problems that affect the lungs include irritation and inflammation accompanied by excess mucus. Some mucus is normal and healthy as it helps to keep the lungs lubricated. However, when the lungs are exposed to allergens, bacteria, viruses or pollutants, mucus production increases.

One of the most damaging pollutants to which the lungs are exposed is tobacco smoke. If you have respiratory problems and you smoke, it is imperative that you stop. Exercise is also very important – long walks in the open-air are ideal. Avoid mucus-forming foods, such as wheat and dairy products, and use herbs, such as basil, chives, garlic, ginger, marjoram, mint, rosemary, savory and thyme in cooking. Drink plenty of fresh juices – they are rich in zinc and vitamin C which boosts the immune system, making the lungs less prone to infection. (N.B. To make a medicinal infusion, steep 1 tablespoon of the dried ingredient in a cup of boiling water for 10 minutes.)

ASTHMA

AN INFLAMMATION AND CONTRACTION OF THE BRONCHI, CAUSING BREATHLESSNESS, WHEEZING, TIGHT CHEST AND COUGHING. ASTHMA MAY BE HEREDITARY. TRIGGERS INCLUDE ALLERGIES, STRESS, EXERCISE AND EXPOSURE TO COLD AIR.

! DO NOT STOP TAKING MEDICATION PRESCRIBED BY YOUR DOCTOR.

✔ Blackcurrant, cabbage, carrot, chervil, grapefruit, honey, horseradish, lettuce, mint, radish, rosemary, savory, sorrel, watercress. Drink chervil, carrot, cabbage, lemon, watercress

and apple juices and infusions of mint, thyme (with lemon juice) and rosemary. During an attack, eat a lump of sugar infused with three drops of fennel essential oil.

✘ Dairy products.

RECIPES *carrot, apple and ginger juice (page 112), cabbage, carrot and celery juice (page 113), lemon-balm and camomile infusion (page 118), ginger infusion (page 119), lettuce-seed decoction (page 120), strawberry-leaf decoction (page 120).*

BRONCHITIS

AN INFLAMMATION OF THE LINING OF THE BRONCHI, RESULTING IN COUGHING, SPUTUM PRODUCTION AND BREATHLESSNESS. MAY BE ACUTE (CAUSED BY VIRUSES AND BACTERIA) OR CHRONIC (DUE TO RECURRENT INFECTIONS, SMOKING OR POLLUTION).

✔ Blackcurrants, borage, carrot, chervil, fig, garlic, grape, honey, horseradish, lettuce, mint, quince, radish, sage, savory, thyme, watercress. Drink infusions of rosemary and borage. SEE ALSO general advice on the care of the respiratory system.

✘ Dairy products, wheat.

RECIPES *almond milk (page 71), carrot, apple and ginger juice (page 112), marjoram infusion (page 117), lemon-balm and camomile infusion (page 118), ginger infusion (page 119), lettuce-seed decoction (page 120), leek syrup (page 124).*

COUGH

A SYMPTOM OF AN INFECTION, INFLAMMATION OR IRRITATION OF THE

THROAT, USUALLY ASSOCIATED WITH A COLD, FLU, BRONCHITIS OR SORE THROAT. SEE ALSO IMMUNE SYSTEM.

! IF THE COUGH IS PERSISTENT, OR IF MUCUS IS SPECKLED WITH BLOOD, SEE A DOCTOR IMMEDIATELY.

✔ *SEE* Asthma, Bronchitis and Sore throat (page 79).

HAY FEVER (ALLERGIC RHINITIS)

AN ALLERGIC REACTION TO POLLEN FROM TREES, FLOWERS OR GRASS, CAUSING SNEEZING, RUNNY NOSE AND ITCHING OF THE EYES, NOSE AND THROAT.

✔ *SEE* general advice on the respiratory system and Asthma.
RECIPES marjoram infusion (page 117), lemon-balm and camomile infusion (page 118), elder and camomile infusion (page 118).

PLEURISY

SEVERE ONE-SIDED CHEST PAIN CAUSED BY AN INFLAMMATION OF THE MEMBRANES SURROUNDING THE LUNGS AS A RESULT OF AN UNDERLYING ILLNESS. PAIN IS WORSE ON BREATHING/COUGHING.

✔ Cabbage, carrot, cherry, chervil, fig, garlic, leek, onion, radish, saffron, watercress. *SEE ALSO* Asthma, Bronchitis.
RECIPES cabbage, carrot and celery juice (page 113), marjoram infusion (page 117), lemon-balm and camomile infusion (page 118), elder and camomile infusion (page 118), cherry-stem decoction (page 119), lettuce-seed decoction (page 120).

PNEUMONIA

AN INFLAMMATION OF THE LUNGS, CAUSED BY A VIRUS OR BACTERIA.

SYMPTOMS INCLUDE BREATHLESSNESS, A COUGH THAT MAY PRODUCE BLOODY SPUTUM, HIGH FEVER AND CHEST PAIN. SEVERE CASES LEAD TO COMPLICATIONS AND MAY BE LIFE THREATENING.

! DO NOT STOP TAKING MEDICATION PRESCRIBED BY YOUR DOCTOR.

✔ Foods rich in vitamin C and zinc plus blackberry, borage, carrot, chervil, clove, fig, garlic, juniper berry, lamb's lettuce, leek, nettle, onion, rosemary, savory, thyme. *SEE ALSO* Asthma, Bronchitis.
RECIPES cherry and apple juice (page 112), cabbage, carrot and celery juice (page 113), green bean and garlic juice (page 113), lettuce and basil juice (page 113), celery and red onion juice (page 113), marjoram infusion (page 117), lemon-balm and camomile infusion (page 118), elder and camomile infusion (page 118), cherry-stem decoction (page 119).

SORE THROAT AND TONSILLITIS

SEE SORE THROAT (PAGE 79).

WHOOPING COUGH

A HIGHLY CONTAGIOUS BACTERIAL INFECTION, CAUSING SEVERE SPASMODIC COUGH. OCCURS PRIMARILY IN INFANTS.

! ANTIBIOTIC TREATMENT IS REQUIRED IMMEDIATELY.

✔ Take a mixture of lemon juice and honey. *SEE ALSO* Asthma, Bronchitis and Immune system.
RECIPES almond milk (page 71), marjoram infusion (page 117), lemon-balm and camomile infusion (page 118), elder and camomile infusion (page 118), leek syrup (page 124), black radish syrup (page 124).

SUGGESTED MENU FOR CHRONIC LUNG DISORDERS

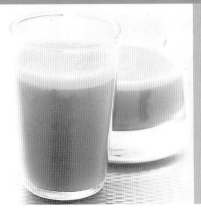

The following menu is designed for someone suffering from a chronic lung disorder such as asthma or bronchitis.

BREAKFAST
A bowl of rice cereal with soya milk; a small glass of carrot juice; a cup of coffee; grapefruit or kiwi fruit.

SNACKS
Dried fruit, especially raisins and figs; fresh fruit, such as orange, kiwi, papaya and pineapple; ginger infusion.

LUNCH
Black radish salad and grilled fish with mustard or horseradish sauce; melon with fresh mint.

DINNER
Red lentil soup (page 89) with rye bread; avocado tartar (page 95); lettuce-seed, marjoram or lemon-balm infusion.

kidneys and bladder

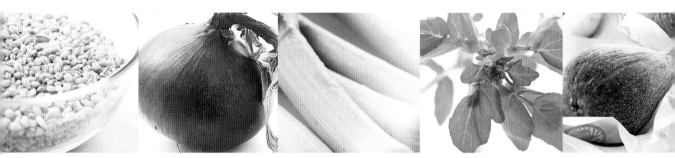

STAR FOODS FOR THE KIDNEYS AND BLADDER: BARLEY, BLACKCURRANT, BLUEBERRY, CABBAGE, CELERY, CRANBERRY, CUCUMBER, DANDELION, FIG, FRESH FRUIT, GRAPE, LEEK, ONION, UNPROCESSED CEREALS, WATERCRESS, WHEATGERM.

The kidneys' role in the body is to filter waste products from the blood. The waste is then eliminated from the body via the bladder and urethra in the form of urine. The body produces approximately one litre of urine daily and the bladder is emptied, on average, four to six times a day. The appearance of your urine provides a rough indication of whether you are drinking enough: a dark orange or amber colour is a sign that you need to increase your fluid intake. Changes in urinary habits or function that warrant medical attention include: cloudy or discoloured urine, unexplained changes in urinary output, and pain or discomfort on urination. A problem that becomes common in men over the age of 50 is enlarged prostate gland (page 83). This typically causes a hesitant, weak or trickling flow of urine from the urethra.

You can enhance your kidney function by drinking more water, fruit juices and herbal infusions, and regularly eating foods from the above list. You should reduce your intake of coffee, tea and alcohol. Alcohol suppresses the production of antidiuretic hormone in the body, dramatically increasing the output of urine by the kidneys. Foods that are rich in fibre and magnesium, such as fresh fruit, unprocessed cereals and wheatgerm, are beneficial to the kidneys and bladder. It is also important to prevent kidney, bladder and urethral infections by keeping your immune system healthy (pages 78–79). (N.B. To make a medicinal infusion, steep 1 tablespoon of the dried ingredient in a cup of boiling water for 10 minutes.)

BLADDER OR KIDNEY STONES

SMALL HARD MASSES OF CALCIUM AND OTHER SALTS OCCURRING ANYWHERE IN THE URINARY TRACT. STONES MAY LODGE IN THE BLADDER CAUSING FREQUENT, PAINFUL URINATION AND BLOOD IN THE URINE; THEY MAY OCCUR IN THE URINE-COLLECTING DUCT OF THE KIDNEYS CAUSING SEVERE PAIN; OR THEY MAY REMAIN IN THE KIDNEYS CAUSING MILD PAIN. KIDNEY OR BLADDER STONES MAY NECESSITATE SURGERY OR ANOTHER MEDICAL PROCEDURE.

! DRINK AT LEAST 6–8 GLASSES OF WATER PER DAY AND 1 DURING THE NIGHT.

✔ Almond, artichoke, bean, blackberry, blackcurrant, broad bean, cabbage, celery, cherry, chickpea, chicory, dandelion, grape, green bean, lamb's lettuce, leek, lettuce, melon, nettle, olive, onion, peach, physalis, radish, redcurrant, strawberry, tomato, watercress. Drink olive-leaf infusion and blackcurrant, grape, cranberry, cherry and watercress juices.

✗ Animal protein, chocolate, coffee, gooseberry, nettle, peanut, rhubarb, sorrel, spinach, tea.

RECIPES broad bean-flower infusion (page 24), chickpea broth (page 86), cabbage, carrot and celery juice (page 113), celery and red onion juice (page 113), cucumber and lettuce heart juice (page 113), physalis jam (page 116), dandelion infusion (page 117), pear and apple infusion (page 118), corn-hair and fennel-seed decoction (page 119), physalis-berry decoction (page 120), strawberry-leaf decoction (page 120), barley water (page 121), juniper-berry wine (page 122).

CYSTITIS AND URETHRITIS

INFLAMMATION OF THE BLADDER AND URETHRA CAUSED BY AN INFECTION. SYMPTOMS INCLUDE PAIN IN THE LOWER ABDOMEN, FREQUENT, URGENT AND PAINFUL URINATION AND BLOOD IN THE URINE. CYSTITIS IS MOST COMMON IN WOMEN.

✔ Artichoke, blueberry, cherry, cranberry, cucumber, dandelion, juniper berry, melon, pumpkin, redcurrant, strawberry, thyme, watermelon. Drink plenty of water and watercress, blackcurrant, blueberry, cranberry and grape juices.

✘ Asparagus.

RECIPES cabbage, carrot and blueberry juice (page 19), chickpea broth (page 86), cherry and raspberry juice (page 112), cherry and apple juice (page 112), cabbage, carrot and celery juice (page 113), celery and red onion juice (page 113), cucumber and lettuce heart juice (page 113), physalis jam (page 116), corn-hair and fennel-seed decoction (page 119), physalis-berry decoction (page 120), strawberry-leaf decoction (page 120), barley water (page 121).

ENLARGED PROSTATE GLAND

THE GLAND GROWS TO THE POINT WHERE IT NARROWS THE URETHRA AND IMPEDES THE FLOW OF URINE. SEE MEN'S HEALTH.

IRRITABLE BLADDER

A FREQUENT URGE TO PASS URINE. SEE CYSTITIS AND URETHRITIS.

PYELONEPHRITIS

AN INFECTION OF THE KIDNEYS (ACUTE OR CHRONIC) CAUSING PAIN IN THE BACK AND LOWER ABDOMEN, FEVER AND PAINFUL URINATION.
! ANTIBIOTICS ARE URGENTLY REQUIRED.

✔ Almond, artichoke, bean, blackberry, blackcurrant, borage, broad bean, cabbage, celery, cherry, chickpea, chicory, cucumber, dandelion, garlic, grape, leek, lettuce, melon, onion, peach, physalis, radish, redcurrant, strawberry, watercress, watermelon. Drink plenty of water as well as onion, cabbage, celery, cucumber, watercress, grape, cranberry, cherry and blueberry juices.

RECIPES cabbage, carrot and blueberry juice (page 19), chickpea broth (page 86), cherry and apple juice (page 112), celery and red onion juice (page 113), cucumber and lettuce heart juice (page 113), physalis jam (page 116), corn-hair and fennel-seed decoction (page 119), physalis-berry decoction (page 120), strawberry-leaf decoction (page 120), barley water (page 121).

SUGGESTED MENUS FOR KIDNEY AND BLADDER PROBLEMS

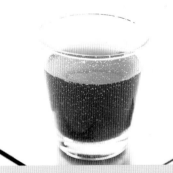

The following menus are designed to enhance the health of the urinary tract for people who are suffering from problems such as kidney or bladder stones. The emphasis is on drinking plenty of fluids and eating foods that have diuretic and anti-inflammatory properties such as chickpea, leek and onion.

MENU 1

BREAKFAST

A bowl of cereal or porridge; a small glass of celery and carrot juice; a cup of herbal tea; grapefruit or kiwi fruit.

SNACKS

Dried fruit, such as fig, or fresh fruit rich in vitamin C, such as orange; dandelion or ginger infusion; cranberry juice.

LUNCH

Courgette cake (page 97) and grilled fish with rice and cucumber; barley water (page 121); melon with fresh mint.

DINNER

Buckwheat with leek sauce (page 97); blueberries and cottage cheese (page 35); lettuce seed or thyme infusion; juniper decoction.

MENU 2

BREAKFAST

A boiled egg with rye bread; a juice (celery and onion, or green bean, lettuce and garlic); live yoghurt; a cup of herbal tea.

SNACKS

Dried fruit, especially raisin and fig; fresh fruit, such as blackcurrant, blueberry and pear; barley water (page 121).

LUNCH

Onions in cider (page 103) with a slice of roast meat, bread and a little table mustard; a cucumber salad; a piece of fruit.

DINNER

Chickpea broth (page 86) with bread; barley water (page 121); thyme or camomile infusion.

nervous system, mind and emotions

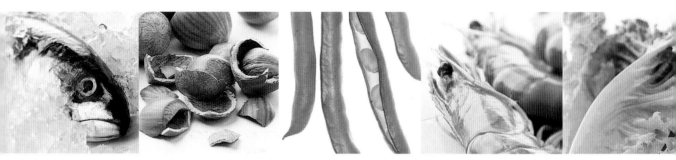

STAR FOODS FOR THE NERVOUS SYSTEM: APPLE, APRICOT, ASPARAGUS, AVOCADO, BANANA, BEETROOT, CABBAGE, CAMOMILE, CELERY, DILL SEED, FISH, GREEN VEGETABLES, LETTUCE, NUTS, OAT, PEACH, PULSES, PUMPKIN, QUINCE, POTATO, SHELLFISH, UNREFINED CEREALS.

Good stress management, relaxation, meditation and open-air exercise combined with small dietary changes can alleviate many symptoms of common nervous system disorders. Foods that have a calming effect on the nervous system are those that are rich in vitamin B, folic acid, magnesium, potassium, zinc, selenium and manganese. Try to eat plenty of fish, green vegetables, nuts, potatoes, pulses and unrefined cereals. Increase your intake of proteins and cut down on alcohol, coffee and tea. Drink infusions of camomile, lemon verbena, lemon balm, limeflower, olive-tree leaf, orange blossom or valerian. Bear in mind that problems such as irritability and poor concentration – as well as headaches and dizziness – may be caused by mild hypoglycaemia, in which case you should eat regular carbohydrate-based meals or snacks. (N.B. To make a medicinal infusion, steep 1 tablespoon of the dried ingredient in a cup of boiling water for 10 minutes.)

ANXIETY

PSYCHOLOGICAL SYMPTOMS SUCH AS FEAR ARE ASSOCIATED WITH TENSION, SWEATING, PALPITATIONS, INSOMNIA AND LOSS OF APPETITE.

✔ Almond, apple, apricot, aubergine, basil, bean, beetroot, celery, lemon balm, lettuce, peach, pulses, quince. Drink fresh apple,

apricot, cucumber, lettuce or peach juices and aniseed, basil, camomile, lemon-balm, lettuce-seed, limeflower, rosemary or thyme infusions. Eat more carbohydrates. Eating sugary snacks may reduce anxiety – this should be an occasional measure only.

✘ Coffee, cola drinks, tea.

RECIPES *lemon-balm and camomile infusion (page 118), sparkling lemon-balm infusion (page 119), lettuce-seed decoction (page 120), camomile and citrus wine (page 123), asparagus syrup (page 125).*

DEPRESSION

A NEGATIVE MENTAL STATE ASSOCIATED WITH A BROAD SPECTRUM OF PHYSICAL SYMPTOMS.

✔ Oats, walnuts, fresh fruit and vegetables that are rich in vitamin B complex. SEE ALSO Anxiety.

✘ Alcohol.

HEADACHES AND MIGRAINE

OFTEN CAUSED BY LOCAL MUSCLE TENSION OR STRESS; MIGRAINES ARE SEVERE, PROLONGED HEADACHES THAT MAY BE TRIGGERED BY CERTAIN FOODS, HORMONAL FLUCTUATIONS OR HYPOGLYCAEMIA.

✔ Almond, anise, basil, broad bean, cabbage, camomile, cherry, chive, fennel, ginger, lemon balm, mint, oily fish, onion, peach, rosemary, white meat. Eat plenty of fresh fruit and vegetables. Drink fresh apple, apricot and lettuce juices or aniseed, basil, camomile, fennel-seed, lemon-balm or mint infusions. *SEE ALSO* Anxiety.

✗ Alcohol, coffee, cheese, chocolate, food with additives ("E" numbers), ice-cream, monosodium glutamate, sweeteners, tea. *RECIPES ginger infusion (page 119), basil liqueur (page 123), anisette (page 123), aniseed tincture (page 124).*

INSOMNIA

A PATTERN OF PERSISTENT SHORT SLEEPING, EITHER WITH DIFFICULTY FALLING ASLEEP OR FREQUENTLY INTERRUPTED SLEEP.

✔ Aubergine, basil, barley, camomile, corn, courgette, fennel, lettuce, lime blossom, marjoram, onion, pumpkin. Eat a carbohydrate snack 20 minutes before you go to bed. *SEE ALSO* Anxiety.

✗ Coffee, cola drinks, tea.
RECIPES lime-blossom infusion (page 46), mango juice (page 112), marjoram infusion (page 117), lemon-balm and camomile infusion (page 118), sparkling lemon-balm infusion (page 119), camomile and citrus wine (page 123), camomile aperitif (page 123), asparagus syrup (page125).

IRRITABILITY AND STRESS

SYMPTOMS SUCH AS ANXIETY, POOR CONCENTRATION AND INSOMNIA ARE OFTEN COMBINED WITH PHYSICAL SYMPTOMS SUCH AS DIGESTIVE DISTURBANCES AND SOMETIMES HIGH BLOOD PRESSURE.

✔ *SEE* Anxiety, Insomnia, Heart and circulation, Digestive system.

MENTAL FATIGUE

LACK OF MENTAL FOCUS AND POOR CONCENTRATION AND MEMORY.

✔ Fruit and vegetables (especially apricots and carrots), mint, royal jelly, shellfish, foods rich in vitamin B (green vegetables and unrefined cereals), zinc and selenium. Drink apricot, cherry and grape juices and basil and mint infusions. *SEE ALSO* Anxiety, Insomnia.

✗ Excessive amounts of coffee and alcohol.

MULTIPLE SCLEROSIS

CHRONIC DEGENERATIVE DISORDER OF THE NERVOUS SYSTEM.

! DO NOT STOP TAKING MEDICATION PRESCRIBED BY YOUR DOCTOR.

✔ Buckwheat, corn, fresh fruit and vegetables, millet, pulses. Eat more oily fish and cold-pressed vegetable oils, such as sunflower seed and olive oil. Drink fresh apple, apricot, cabbage, grape or lettuce juices or aniseed, basil, camomile, fennel-seed, lemon-balm or mint infusions. Take evening primrose oil daily.

✗ Dairy products, gluten, meat.
RECIPES ginger infusion (page 119).

NEURALGIA

SEE HEADACHES AND MIGRAINE.

VERTIGO

DIZZINESS AND LOSS OF BALANCE, SOMETIMES WITH NAUSEA.

! MAY INDICATE A SERIOUS PROBLEM – CONSULT YOUR DOCTOR.

✔ Basil, fennel, lemon balm, orange, mint, sage, thyme. *SEE ALSO* general advice on the care of the nervous system.

SUGGESTED MENU FOR STRESS-RELATED SYMPTOMS

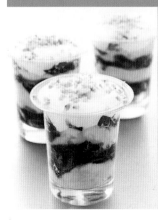

The following menu is designed for someone suffering from mild anxiety, depression, poor concentration, headaches or mild insomnia.

MENU

BREAKFAST

A bowl of porridge; a small glass of carrot juice; herbal infusions such as lemon balm or camomile; a banana.

SNACKS

Dried fruit, such as raisins or figs; fresh fruit rich in vitamin C, such as orange; nuts; herbal infusions.

LUNCH

Grilled meat, beans with carrots and onions (page 104), rice with cucumber balls (page 103) or grated celeriac and carrot salad (page 92); fruit salad with lemon-balm (page 107).

DINNER

Grilled salmon with aubergine sauce (page 97); banana and date salad (page 106); lettuce-seed, camomile or lemon balm infusion.

immune system

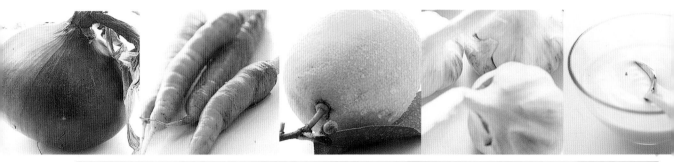

STAR FOODS FOR THE IMMUNE SYSTEM: APPLE, ARTICHOKE, BASIL, BLACKBERRY, BLACKCURRANT, BLUEBERRY, CABBAGE, CAMOMILE, CARROT, CHERRY, CHIVE, CINNAMON, CLOVE, CUCUMBER, CUMIN, DANDELION, ELDER, GARLIC, GREEN BEAN, LEMON, LEMON BALM, LEEK, LIVE YOGHURT, MINT, OILY FISH, PEAR, PULSES, RASPBERRY, RED ONION, REDCURRANT, SHELLFISH, THYME, UNREFINED CEREALS, WATERCRESS, WATERMELON.

The immune system protects the body from infection due to bacteria, viruses and other microbes. Allergies occur when the immune system over-reacts to a substance. Regular physical exercise and a healthy diet strengthen the immune system – poor nutrition, alcohol, drugs and stress weaken it.

To boost your immune system, try to cut down on your intake of alcohol and animal fat and eliminate from your diet any foods that you suspect may be causing an allergy – the most common culprits are citrus fruit, corn, eggs, milk and cheese, nuts, pork, processed tomatoes, shellfish, wheat, and food containing monosodium glutamate or any "E numbers".

Three categories of foods strengthen the immune system:
1) anti-infective: basil, blackberries, blueberries, cinnamon, cloves, cumin, garlic, juniper, lemon, thyme and live yoghurt, which is rich in lactobacilli.
2) anti-inflammatory: apple, artichoke, blackcurrants, cabbage, camomile, cherries, cucumber, elder, lemon balm, mint, oily fish, pears, raspberries, redcurrants, watercress, watermelon.
3) diuretic and depurative: artichoke, chives, dandelion, green beans, leeks, onions.

Green vegetables are rich in vitamins, beta-carotene, minerals and trace elements, all of which play an important part in maintaining a healthy immune system. Red, green and yellow vegetables and fruit contain powerful antioxidants that help prevent the deterioration of the immune system. Oily fish contains an oil that has important anti-inflammatory properties. Fresh raw fruit and vegetables are the best source of vitamin C; and pulses, shellfish and unrefined cereal provide a good supply of zinc, an important immuno-stimulant.
(N.B. To make a medicinal infusion, steep 1 tablespoon of the dried ingredient in a cup of boiling water for 10 minutes.)

CANDIDA

A LOW-LEVEL INFECTION CAUSED BY THE PROLIFERATION OF *CANDIDA ALBICAN*. THIS OCCURS WHEN THE BALANCE OF THE INTESTINAL FLORA IS DISTURBED AFTER TAKING ANTIBIOTICS OR IMMUNO-SUPPRESSANTS.

✔ Blueberry, garlic, live yoghurt, pickled turnip; infusions of cumin seed, thyme, fennel and aniseed. Follow the detox programme on pages 128–31. *SEE ALSO* general advice on the care of the immune system and the digestive system.
RECIPES fennel infusion (page 117), marjoram infusion (page 117).

COMMON COLD

A VIRAL INFECTION CAUSING WATERY DISCHARGE FROM THE NOSE, SLIGHT FEVER, SORE THROAT AND COUGH. RECURRENT COLDS ARE USUALLY A SIGN OF A WEAK IMMUNE SYSTEM.

✔ Basil, blackberry, blueberry, chilli, chive, cinnamon, clove, cumin, garlic, ginger, juniper, lemon, live yoghurt, onion, orange, peppercorns, rosemary, shellfish, spring onion, thyme, unrefined cereal. Eat plenty of fresh, raw fruit and vegetables, especially those that are red, green or yellow in colour. Drink fresh blackberry, carrot, lemon or orange juice.

RECIPES *garlic and sage soup (page 49), chive and ginger broth (page 88), elder and camomile infusion (page 118).*

INFLUENZA

SEE COMMON COLD.

LARYNGITIS

SEE SORE THROAT.

POST-VIRAL FATIGUE

CHRONIC ILLNESS CHARACTERIZED BY LOW ENERGY LEVELS AND POOR CONCENTRATION. USUALLY FOLLOWS A VIRAL ILLNESS.

✔ Fresh apricot, beetroot, blueberry, cabbage, carrot, cherry or grape juices and basil, mint or thyme infusions. SEE ALSO Anaemia (page 63), Mental fatigue (page 77), general advice on the care of the immune system and detoxification (pages 128–31).

RECIPES *garlic tincture (page 48).*

SINUSITIS

AN INFLAMMATION OF THE SINUSES, CAUSED BY RECURRENT COLDS OR FOLLOWING AN UPPER RESPIRATORY TRACT INFECTION. CHRONIC SINUSITIS IS USUALLY CAUSED BY AN ALLERGY. SEE COMMON COLD.

SORE THROAT

A COMMON SYMPTOM RESULTING FROM COLDS, LARYNGITIS, PHARYNGITIS OR TONSILLITIS.

✔ Bay leaf, blackberry, blackcurrant, blueberry, borage, carrot, celery, chervil, clove, fig, garlic, honey, juniper berry, lamb's lettuce, leek, lemon, onion, peppercorns, nettle, rosemary, savory, thyme, vinegar. SEE ALSO general advice on the care of the immune system and the respiratory system.

RECIPES *almond milk (page 71), marjoram infusion (page 117), leek syrup (page 124), black radish syrup (page 124).*

TONSILLITIS

AN ACUTE INFLAMMATION OF THE TONSILS, MOST FREQUENT IN CHILDREN.

✔ A thyme infusion with honey and lemon juice may help to soothe the pain. SEE ALSO Common cold, Influenza, Sore throat.

RECIPES *redcurrant, blackberry and blueberry juice (page 112), leek syrup (page 124), black radish syrup (page 124).*

SUGGESTED MENUS FOR THE IMMUNE SYSTEM

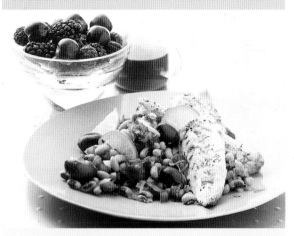

The following menus are designed to enhance the health of the immune system and prevent illness.

MENU 1

BREAKFAST

Live yoghurt with kiwi fruit; a small glass of carrot juice; a cup of dandelion root coffee or a herbal infusion such as lemon balm or camomile.

SNACKS

Fresh fruit rich in vitamin C; nuts; herbal infusions.

LUNCH

Grated celeriac and carrot salad (page 92); dandelion, bacon and potato cakes (page 100); lychee fruit salad (page 106).

DINNER

Spinach with green beans; camomile or lemon balm infusion.

MENU 2

BREAKFAST

A boiled egg with wholemeal bread; a glass of carrot juice.

SNACKS

Dried fruit or nuts; dandelion infusion.

LUNCH

Mediterranean bean salad (page 90); boiled fish; fruit salad.

DINNER

Nettle or watercress soup (page 88); cottage cheese with blueberries (page 35); elderflower and camomile infusion.

skin, hair and nails

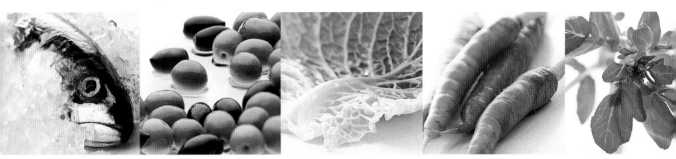

STAR FOODS FOR SKIN, HAIR AND NAILS: ALL RED, YELLOW OR GREEN FRUIT AND VEGETABLES, CABBAGE, CAMOMILE, CARROT, CHERVIL, DANDELION, OILY FISH, OLIVE, SHELLFISH, WATERCRESS.

To improve or control a skin condition, try following a detox programme (see pages 128–31). Try to identify any foods to which you may be allergic and to eliminate them from your diet. If you smoke, make an effort to give up. Treat the skin externally by applying skin washes and poultices to eliminate inflammation and bacterial activity (see specific skin problems).

The following foods promote healthy skin, hair and nails:
1) dandelion is a general detoxifier;
2) carrots and all red, yellow or green fruit and vegetables are rich in beta-carotene and antioxidants;
3) green, leafy vegetables contain vitamins and minerals that are beneficial for the skin;
4) camomile infusion can help to relieve stress (which may exacerbate skin problems), it can also be used as a skin wash;
5) shellfish and oily fish contain essential fatty acids and minerals. (N.B. To make a medicinal infusion, steep 1 tablespoon of the dried ingredient in a cup of boiling water for 10 minutes.)

ACNE

A SKIN CONDITION CHARACTERIZED BY INFLAMED SPOTS ON THE FACE, NECK OR BACK, USUALLY RELATED TO HORMONAL FLUCTUATIONS.

✔ Foods that are rich in zinc and vitamin A. Apply cabbage leaves or juice, carrot juice or a lettuce-seed decoction to very inflamed spots and use a camomile infusion as a face wash.

✘ Cheese, chocolate, food that is rich in iodine (such as shellfish and kelp), refined carbohydrate.

RECIPES cabbage, carrot and blueberry juice (page 19), juniper-berry water (apply externally, see page 51), black radish and carrot juice (page 113).

BOILS AND CARBUNCLES

SEE ACNE.

DANDRUFF

A FLAKY SCALP, SOMETIMES CAUSED BY A YEAST INFECTION.

✔ After washing, rinse your hair thoroughly with a thyme or rosemary infusion.

SEE ALSO general advice on the care of the Skin, hair and nails.

DERMATITIS AND ECZEMA

AN INFLAMMATION OF THE SKIN WHICH IS OFTEN CHRONIC. SORES MAY BE DRY AND ITCHY OR WEEPING.

✔ Artichoke, carrot, chervil, cucumber, dandelion, all green vegetables, grape, melon, oily fish, raspberry, salsify. An application of olive or walnut oil is effective in relieving dry skin. A camomile or thyme infusion can be used as a skin wash to reduce inflammation and prevent bacterial activity.

✘ Alcohol and spicy food. Reduce your intake of dairy products, meat, processed food and any other suspected allergens.

RECIPES cabbage, carrot and blueberry juice (page 19), juniper-berry water (apply externally, see page 51), black radish and carrot juice (page 113), dandelion infusion (page 117).

FUNGAL INFECTIONS

AN IRRITATION OF THE SKIN BETWEEN THE TOES OR FINGERS, AROUND
THE GROIN OR ON THE SCALP.

✔ Use a thyme infusion to bathe or wash the affected area. *SEE
ALSO* general care of the Immune system.

PSORIASIS

A HEREDITARY CONDITION CAUSING AN EXCESSIVE PRODUCTION
OF NEW SKIN CELLS. THIS RESULTS IN SORE, SCALY PATCHES ON
THE SKIN.

! STRESS IS KNOWN TO AGGRAVATE AND EVEN TRIGGER PSORIASIS.

✔ Eat plenty of oily fish and increase your exposure to sunlight. *SEE
ALSO* Irritability and stress (page 77).

✘ Animal fat and dairy products.

ROSACEA

A CHRONIC INFLAMMATION OF THE FACE CAUSING RED AREAS TO
APPEAR ON THE CHEEKS, NOSE, FOREHEAD AND CHIN.

! THE CONDITION IS EXACERBATED BY ALCOHOL AND STRESS.

✔ Try following a dairy-free diet. Use a camomile infusion as an
anti-inflammatory face wash. A thyme infusion or cabbage or
lettuce leaves applied to the affected area can also help to reduce
the inflammation.

✘ Alcohol and spicy food.

RECIPES cabbage, carrot and blueberry juice (page 19), black-radish
and carrot juice (page 113).

URTICARIA (HIVES)

RAISED RED, ITCHY PATCHES CAUSE BY AN ALLERGIC REACTION AND
AGGRAVATED BY STRESS.

! THIS CONDITION MAY BE A REACTION TO A PRESCRIPTION DRUG –
CONSULT YOUR DOCTOR. HIVES CAN BE DANGEROUS IF THE MOUTH,
LIPS AND TONGUE ARE AFFECTED.

✔ Artichoke, carrot, cucumber, dandelion, green vegetables
(especially nettle and watercress), radish, watermelon. Drink
camomile or lemon-balm infusions. Use a mixture of equal
amounts of camomile and peppermint infusion as a skin wash.

✘ Try to identify and eliminate the cause of the allergy (for example
strawberries or shellfish). Avoid alcohol, animal fat, dairy products,
eggs, stimulants and wheat for a few days.

RECIPES lemon-balm and camomile infusion (page 118), sparkling
lemon-balm infusion (page 119).

women's, health

For specific conditions affecting women's health, see below.
For lactating mothers, fennel is recommended, as it is thought
to stimulate the baby's appetite and prevent colic and digestive
problems; dill enhances the flavour of breast milk.
(N.B. To make a medicinal infusion, steep 1 tablespoon of the
dried ingredient in a cup of boiling water for 10 minutes.)

AMENORRHOEA

ABSENCE OF OR IRREGULAR PERIODS. MAY BE CAUSED BY HORMONAL
IMBALANCE, STRESS, OVER-EXERCISE, RAPID WEIGHT LOSS OR
ANOREXIA.

✔ Anise, dill, dried fruit, fennel, green, leafy vegetables, liver,
parsley, red meat, sage, yeast extract. Drink fresh apricot, broccoli
or spinach juice and aniseed, fennel-seed or sage infusion.
RECIPES apricot, lime and mint juice (page 111), broccoli and green-
bean juice (page 113), fennel infusion (page 117), carrot seed
infusion (page 118), coriander-seed infusion (page 119), corn-hair
and fennel-seed decoction (page 119), dill-seed decoction (page
120), fennel-seed decoction (page 120), anisette (page 123),
aniseed tincture (page 124), coriander-seed tincture (page 124).

CYSTITIS

SEE KIDNEYS AND BLADDER.

DIGESTIVE PROBLEMS DURING PREGNANCY

PROBLEMS SUCH AS HEARTBURN, SLUGGISH DIGESTION, HYPER-
ACIDITY AND INDIGESTION ARE COMMON DURING PREGNANCY.

✔ Apple, banana, carrot, courgette, fig, germinated barley, ginger,
papaya, peach, pineapple, potato. Eat small, frequent meals. Drink
apple, carrot, peach or pineapple juice; and basil, camomile, fennel-
seed or lemon-balm infusion. *SEE ALSO* constipation (page 68).

✘ Avoid fatty and processed foods.

RECIPES fennel infusion (page 117), lemon-balm and camomile
infusion (page 118), corn-hair and fennel-seed decoction

(page 119), sparkling lemon-balm infusion (page 119), ginger infusion (page 119), fennel-seed decoction (page 120), barley water (page 121).

ENDOMETRIOSIS

INFLAMMATION RESULTING FROM FRAGMENTS OF THE ENDOMETRIUM MIGRATING IN THE PELVIS AND AROUND THE INTESTINES CAUSING PAINFUL PERIODS AND SHARP PAIN IN THE PELVIS DURING INTERCOURSE. SEE PREMENSTRUAL SYNDROME AND PAINFUL PERIODS.

FLUID RETENTION

SOME WOMEN SUFFER FROM FLUID RETENTION PRIOR TO MENSTRUATION OR DURING PREGNANCY.

✔ Drink barley infusion. Leek and onion are good diuretics.

RECIPES barley infusion (page 118)

IRREGULAR PERIODS

SEE AMENORRHOEA.

MENOPAUSAL SYMPTOMS

THE HORMONAL CHANGES ASSOCIATED WITH THE MENOPAUSE (CESSATION OF PERIODS AROUND THE AGE OF 50) GIVE RISE TO A RANGE OF SYMPTOMS INCLUDING HOT FLUSHES AND MOOD SWINGS.

✔ Foods rich in calcium and manganese: avocado, cottage cheese, chestnut, date, fig, green vegetables, live yoghurt, nut, soya, tea, tofu, unrefined cereals. Foods rich in boron: almond, raisin, prune, soya. Food rich in B vitamins (pages 132–3). Drink fresh cabbage, cherry, grape, grapefruit and watercress juice and aniseed, camomile, cumin-seed, lemon-balm and sage infusion and live yoghurt drinks.

RECIPES cabbage, carrot and blueberry juice (page 19), cherry and apple juice (page 112), cherry and raspberry juice (page 112), lemon-balm and camomile infusion (page 118), sparkling lemon-balm infusion (page 119), cumin-seed decoction (page 120), anisette (page 123), aniseed tincture (page 124).

MORNING SICKNESS

NAUSEA, AND SOMETIMES VOMITING, IS A COMMON SYMPTOM IN THE FIRST TRIMESTER OF PREGNANCY.

✔ Eat small, frequent meals and increase your intake of carbohydrate (bean, bread, chestnut, pasta and rice). Drinking fennel, ginger or peppermint infusions or a eating a small amount of crystallized ginger can help alleviate nausea.

RECIPES fennel infusion (page 117), ginger infusion (page 119).

PERIOD PAIN

PAIN IN THE LOWER ABDOMEN JUST BEFORE AND DURING PERIODS.

✔ Aniseed, dill and sage have hormone-like properties – drink as infusions. The following are powerful antispasmodics and analgesics and are excellent as infusions for abdominal cramps and pain: bay leaf, camomile, chive and spring onion, coriander seed, fennel, mint, onion and shallot, rosemary, saffron, tarragon.

RECIPES tarragon-infused oil (apply externally, see page 44), raspberry-leaf infusion (page 117), lemon-balm and camomile infusion (page 118), coriander-seed infusion (page 119), dill-seed decoction (page 120).

PREGNANCY (GENERAL WELL-BEING)

GOOD NUTRITION IS IMPORTANT FOR THE HEALTH OF BOTH MOTHER AND BABY DURING PREGNANCY.

✔ Foods that are rich in iron and folic acid (these include dried fruit and dark-green, leafy vegetables such as watercress, spinach and broccoli) should be eaten on a daily basis, plus beetroot, blackberry, celery, fennel root, germinated pulses, live yoghurt, red meat, unrefined cereals. Drink one and a half litres of mineral water every day and fresh apple, apricot, beetroot, cabbage, grape, green-bean, lettuce or watercress juice and camomile, fennel, lime-blossom flower and mint infusion.

✘ Alcohol and fast or processed food. Do not smoke.

RECIPES cabbage, carrot and blueberry juice (page 19), apple and raspberry juice (page 111), apricot, lime and mint juice (page 111), cherry and apple juice (page 112), green-bean and garlic juice (page 113), beetroot and celery juice (page 113), lettuce and basil juice (page 113), fennel infusion (page 117), raspberry-leaf infusion (page 117), lemon-balm and camomile infusion (page 118), ginger infusion (page 119), fennel-seed decoction (page 120).

PREMENSTRUAL SYNDROME (PMS)

A VARIETY OF PHYSICAL AND EMOTIONAL SYMPTOMS OCCURRING A FEW DAYS BEFORE A PERIOD IS DUE. SYMPTOMS INCLUDE CONSTIPATION, FATIGUE, FLUID RETENTION, IRRITABILITY, LOWER ABDOMINAL PAIN AND DISTENSION, AND MOOD SWINGS.

✔ Increase your intake of fruit and vegetables rich in vitamin B6, calcium, magnesium, manganese and zinc (pages 134–5). Eat small, frequent meals rich in carbohydrates (bean, bread, chestnut, pasta and rice) and root vegetables. Aniseed, dill and sage have hormone-like properties – drink as infusions; tarragon and mint are powerful anti-spasmodics and analgesics and are excellent as infusions for abdominal cramps. Barley contains an amino acid that may help to relieve PMS. SEE ALSO general advice on the care of the Nervous system, and Irritability and stress (page 77).

✘ Fatty or salty foods, stimulants such as coffee, cola drinks and tea. Reduce your consumption of dairy products.

RECIPES *celery and red onion juice (page 113), cucumber and lettuce heart juice (page 113), lettuce and basil juice (page 113), lemon-balm and camomile infusion (page 118), sparkling lemon-balm infusion (page 119).*

THRUSH

A VAGINAL INFECTION RESULTING IN SORENESS AND DISCHARGE. SEE CANDIDA (PAGE 78). DOUCHE WITH CAMOMILE AND THYME INFUSION.

men's health

ENLARGED PROSTATE

A COMMON CONDITION IN MEN OVER 45. DIFFICULTY URINATING IN THE MORNING IS AN EARLY SYMPTOM OF AN ENLARGED PROSTRATE.

✔ Bread, chicken, corn, dried fig, egg, fish, green vegetables, live yoghurt, nettle, nut, pumpkin seed, pumpkin seed oil, soya, tofu and foods rich in zinc (page 135). The following remedy may alleviate the condition: mix equal amounts of almond, brazil nut, cucumber seed, linseed, peanut, pumpkin seed, sesame seed, soya bean and walnut. Make into a paste using a food processor. Take 2 tablespoons daily.

PROSTATITIS

SEE ENLARGED PROSTATE AND GENERAL ADVICE ON THE CARE OF THE IMMUNE SYSTEM.

✔ Infusions of juniper berries or blueberries.

children's health

Most of the advice given in this part of the book also applies to children, with the exception of alcohol-based preparations.

ANXIETY, FEAR, NIGHTMARES

✔ Infusions of camomile, lemon balm or linden in the evening.

RECIPES *lemon-balm and camomile infusion (page 118), sparkling lemon-balm infusion (page 119).*

CHICKENPOX

SEE MEASLES.

CONSTIPATION

SEE DIGESTIVE SYSTEM.

✔ For infants, use puréed boiled carrot or cooked apple.

RECIPES *peach syrup (page 124).*

DIARRHOEA

SEE DIGESTIVE SYSTEM.

✔ Blueberry, boiled carrot and rice water (see Rice; page 27) are the safest dietary remedies for children.

MEASLES

A HIGHLY CONTAGIOUS VIRAL INFECTION CHARACTERIZED BY FEVER AND A SKIN RASH.

✔ Blackberry, celery, cherry, cucumber, onion and thyme help reduce fever and fight infection. Camomile tea can be used as a skin wash to calm down itching and irritation. Olive oil mixed with 3 per cent of lavender essential oil is also helpful for skin rashes.

RECIPES *cabbage, carrot and blueberry juice (page 19), black-radish and carrot juice (page 113), cherry-stem decoction (page 119), cherry-stem and apple decoction (page 120).*

WHOOPING COUGH

SEE RESPIRATORY SYSTEM.

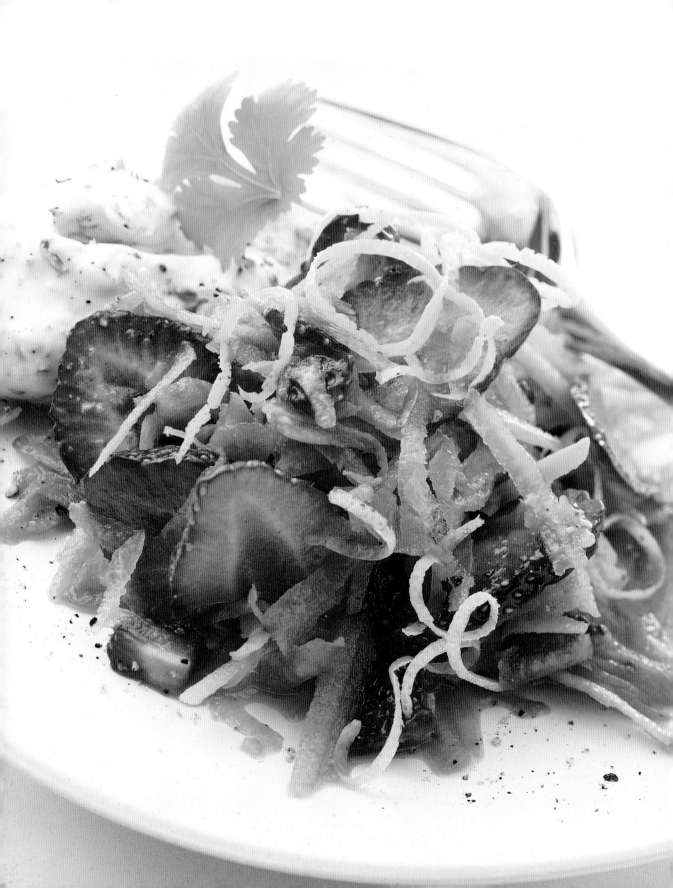

part three

healing
recipes

Incorporating medicinal foods into our diet is a perfect opportunity for creative and delicious cooking. The recipes on the following pages range from quick and unusual dishes that boost good health to recipes for medicinal drinks, tinctures and syrups that target specific ailments (bear in mind that some of the wines and liqueurs need to be prepared in advance). To find ways of using a particular medicinal food, start with the food – by looking in part one of the book where you will find references to the recipes in this section. To find a dish or a remedy that will alleviate a particular ailment, start with the ailment – by looking under the appropriate body system in part two where beneficial recipes are recommended. Or simply browse through the recipes to devise your own health-giving menu.

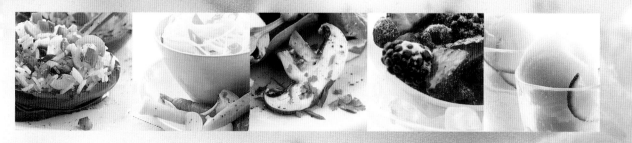

soups and salads

The following recipes serve 4 people unless otherwise stated. Where possible, harvest your own ingredients or use fresh, organic produce. Take care to wash ingredients thoroughly.

SOUPS

croutons

1 clove of garlic
4 thick slices of bread, 1 day old at least
Olive oil

Rub the garlic on the bread, then dice the bread and fry lightly in olive oil. Leave to drain on kitchen paper for a few minutes.

broad bean soup *(right)*

1½ kg fresh or dried broad beans
2 tablespoons olive oil
1 red onion, finely chopped
50 g fresh chervil, parsley or rocket, chopped
2 litres cold water
Salt and pepper
To serve: croutons (recipe above)

Soak the dried broad beans according to the instructions on the packet. In a saucepan, heat the olive oil and add the onion. Cover and sweat slowly for 10 minutes over a gentle heat. Add the broad beans, chervil and water. Bring to the boil and simmer until the beans are cooked. Blend the soup in a food processor, add salt and pepper and serve hot with croutons.

herbal broth

50 g sorrel leaves, finely chopped
25 g lettuce leaves, finely chopped
25 g Swiss chard leaves, finely chopped
25 g fresh chervil, finely chopped
25 g leeks, chopped
Salt to taste
1½ litres water
1 tablespoon olive oil

Blend all the ingredients in a food processor. Transfer the mixture to a saucepan. Bring to the boil, and then simmer for 20 minutes or until cooked.

borscht

½ medium green or white cabbage
½ medium red cabbage
2 medium red beetroots, peeled
1½ litres stock (meat or vegetable)
1 parsnip, peeled and cut in two
1 large carrot, peeled and cut in two
A few cumin seeds
3 tablespoons tomato purée
2 tablespoons red wine vinegar
Salt and pepper
To serve: soured cream or yoghurt

Chop the cabbage and one of the beetroots into thin strips. In a large saucepan, bring the stock to the boil and add the cabbage, beetroot strips, parsnip, carrot, cumin and tomato purée. Cover and simmer for approximately 1 hour, topping up with stock if necessary. Remove the parsnip and carrot from the broth (if they have not already disintegrated), mash with a fork and return to the saucepan. Using a juicer, extract the juice from the remaining beetroot. Add the juice, vinegar, salt and pepper to the broth. Serve with a little soured cream or yoghurt.

chickpea broth

Boiling chickpeas and barley together produces a medicinal decoction that has diuretic properties and can be drunk as a treatment for cystitis and oedema. Simply drain off the cooking water after 30 minutes and store in the refrigerator. Top up the pan with water and continue cooking. The finished broth is bland in taste and excellent for babies or people recovering from illness.

100 g chickpeas, soaked and allowed to germinate (this may take up to 48 hours)
150 g pot barley
1 litre water
Salt and pepper
50 g fresh parsley, chopped

Boil the chickpeas and the barley in the water for 60 minutes or until thoroughly cooked. Season with salt and pepper. Add the parsley and leave to infuse for 10 minutes. Blend in a food processor and serve.

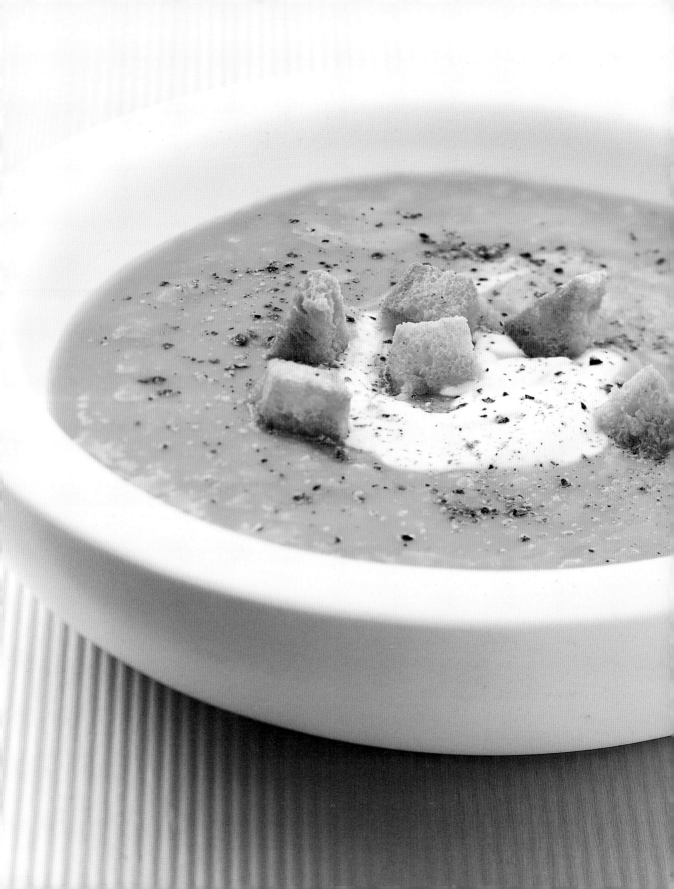

chive and ginger broth *(below)*

1 bunch of chives or 8 spring onions, trimmed
1 clove
5-cm piece root ginger, peeled and sliced
2 cloves of garlic
5 black peppercorns
Small root of Chinese angelica, chopped
1 litre water

Boil all the ingredients in the water for 15 minutes and serve hot. Chicken pieces can be added to this broth – put the raw pieces in the broth and simmer for 30 minutes.

nettle soup

Harvest fresh, young nettle tops from nettles growing away from busy paths and polluted areas.

500 g potatoes, peeled and chopped
300 g nettle tops (leaves and stems)
Salt and pepper
75 ml olive oil
2 tablespoons finely chopped fresh chervil or parsley
To serve: croutons (see page 86)

In a large pan, cover the potatoes with cold water. Bring to the boil and then simmer for about 20 minutes or until cooked. Add the nettles and simmer for 5-8 minutes. Season with salt and pepper. In a food processor, blend the soup, then stir in the olive oil and chervil or parsley. Serve hot with croutons.

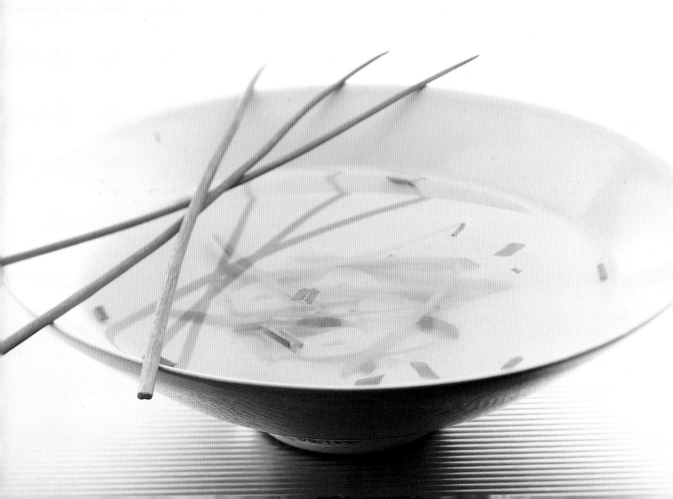

red lentil soup

You can use germinated lentils for this recipe. Buy whole lentils that are green on the outside and red inside rather than split red lentils. Soak them in cold water for 24 hours, then strain, rinse with cold water and place in a flat dish. Cover the lentils with a wet cloth and leave them in a well-ventilated place for a further 24 hours to allow the shoots to grow. Leave the lentils for 48 hours for even longer shoots.

400 g germinated lentils or non-germinated split red lentils
Chicken or vegetable stock (enough to cover the lentils)
3 red onions, chopped
2 tomatoes, chopped
4 cloves of garlic, crushed
2 tablespoons dill
Pepper
A little soured cream, cottage cheese or yoghurt

Steam the lentils for 20 minutes and then cover with chicken or vegetable stock and simmer for a further 20 minutes. Meanwhile, steam the onions, tomatoes and garlic for 5 minutes and then blend in a food processor. Add the onion mixture to the simmering lentils, together with the dill and pepper. Simmer for a further 5 minutes; serve immediately with a little soured cream, cottage cheese or yoghurt.

SALADS

vinaigrette dressing

1 or 2 cloves of garlic (or to taste)
2 tablespoons lemon juice
4 tablespoons olive oil
1 teaspoon Dijon mustard (optional)
Salt and pepper

Crush the garlic, mix with the lemon juice and then stir in the olive oil and mustard if using. Season with salt and pepper and then pour the dressing over the salad. Vinaigrette can be made very quickly by blending the ingredients in a food processor.

avocado dressing

2 avocados, peeled and stoned
1 clove of garlic (optional)
Lemon juice to taste
1 tablespoon Dijon mustard
1 tablespoon finely chopped fresh parsley
Salt and pepper

Blend the ingredients in a food processor and use as an alternative to mayonnaise or vinaigrette.

pepper and aubergine salad

1 green pepper, halved
1 red pepper, halved
1 yellow pepper, halved
500 g aubergine, chopped in small pieces
Salt
Juice of half a lemon
2 shallots, finely chopped
250 g tomatoes, quartered
Vinaigrette dressing
2 tablespoons finely chopped fresh basil or mint

Under a preheated grill, char the peppers. When the skin has turned black put the peppers in a plastic bag and seal it. When cool enough to handle, rub off the skin and slice the peppers thinly. Lightly cook the aubergine in salted, boiling water with the lemon juice until tender. Drain the aubergine and mix with the peppers, shallots and tomatoes. Toss in the vinaigrette and sprinkle with the basil or mint. Chill in the refrigerator for 2 hours before serving.

carrot and strawberry salad

This salad goes well with coriander dressing.

3 tablespoons olive oil
Juice of 1 small lemon
500 g carrot, peeled and grated
300 g strawberries, chopped
Thin strips of lemon zest
To garnish: 3 strawberries

Mix the olive oil and lemon juice in a bowl. Add the carrots and strawberries. Garnish with the 3 strawberries and the lemon zest. This salad will improve if it is refrigerated for 3 hours.

coriander dressing

1 tablespoon finely chopped coriander
2 x 150 ml pots live natural yoghurt
Salt and pepper

Mix the coriander with the yoghurt, season with salt and pepper.

mediterranean bean salad *(below)*

200 g dried haricot, borlotti or black-eye beans
Pinch of ground cinnamon
1 onion, finely chopped
2 tomatoes, chopped
50 g black olives
1 clove
Salt and pepper
4 tablespoons olive oil
1 tablespoon chopped fresh mint leaves
To serve: garlic bread

Soak the beans according to the instructions on the packet, then put them in cold water, bring to the boil and simmer for about 2 hours with the cinnamon. Drain the beans and mix them with all the other ingredients, except the mint leaves. Finally, sprinkle the chopped mint leaves on top of the salad and refrigerate for as long as possible (up to 12 hours). Serve with garlic bread.

radish and kumquat salad *(below right)*

Large bunch of radishes, tops removed
2 oranges
12 kumquats
Lemon juice to taste
Pinch of salt
Sugar or clear honey to taste (optional)

Slice the radishes and oranges and mix in a salad bowl. Slice the kumquats in half lengthways and add to bowl. Sprinkle on a little lemon juice and salt. Refrigerate and toss before serving. Sugar or honey can be added to taste.

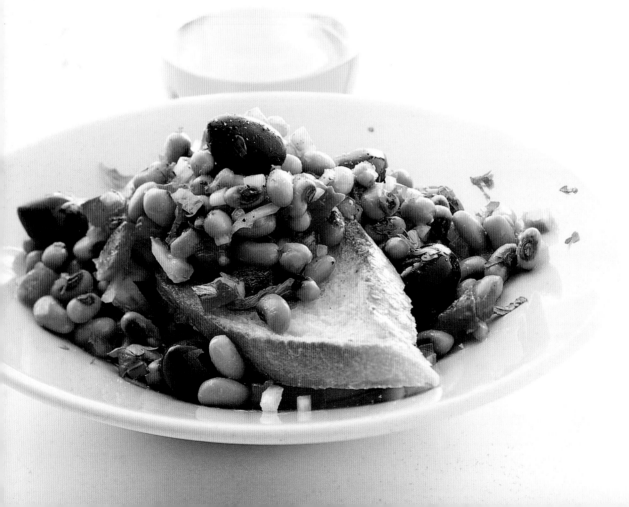

fennel and radicchio salad

2 fennel bulbs, finely chopped
Radicchio leaves (roughly equal in quantity to the fennel)
4 tablespoons vinaigrette (made from one third vinegar or lemon juice
    and two thirds olive oil)

Mix the fennel and radicchio leaves in a large salad bowl. Sprinkle with vinaigrette immediately prior to serving.

green bean salad

500 g green beans
30 g hazelnuts, chopped
3 tablespoons vinaigrette dressing (page 89)
½ lettuce
2 tablespoons chopped fresh parsley or chervil

In boiling, salted water cook the green beans until al dente. When they are ready, plunge them into cold water, then drain. Roast the hazelnuts in a frying pan without oil. Toss the beans in the vinaigrette and place them on a bed of lettuce. Sprinkle the hazelnuts, together with the parsley, over the beans.

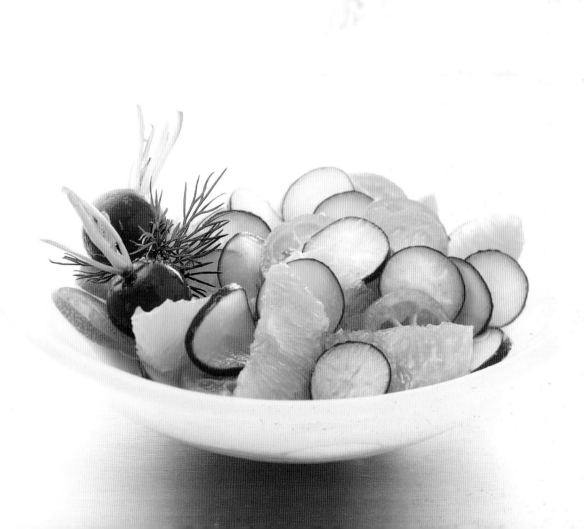

grated celeriac and carrot salad

300 g celeriac, peeled and grated or cut into matchsticks
300 g carrots, peeled and grated or cut into matchsticks
A few tablespoons avocado dressing (page 89)
2 tablespoons finely chopped fresh chervil or parsley

In boiling, salted water blanch the celeriac for 5 seconds and drain. Mix together the celeriac and raw carrot and toss in the mayonnaise (use just enough to coat the vegetables). Refrigerate for 2 hours, garnish with the chervil or parsley and serve.

young turnip salad *(below)*

This salad goes well with thin slices of smoked fish.

1 kg young turnips, peeled
½ litre chicken or vegetable stock
3 tablespoons finely chopped fresh chives
3 tablespoons finely chopped fresh tarragon
3 tablespoons finely chopped fresh chervil
2 tablespoons olive oil
1 tablespoon lemon juice

In boiling, salted water blanch the turnips for 2 minutes. Drain and then cook further in the stock for 10–15 minutes. Drain and allow to cool. Place the turnips in a serving dish and sprinkle over the chives, tarragon and chervil. Mix the olive oil and lemon juice together and pour over the turnips. Gently toss the salad and serve warm.

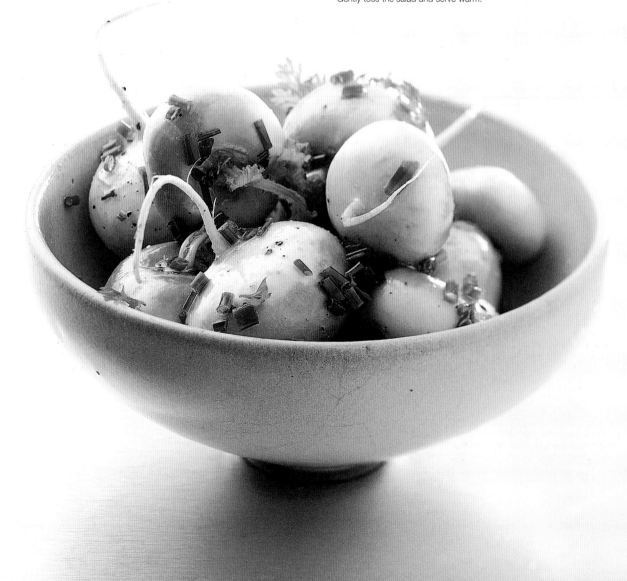

escarole salad

1 escarole (or any type of salad leaf)
A few radishes, tops removed
100 g black olives, stoned
A few anchovies (optional)
3 tomatoes, quartered
1 shallot, finely chopped
2 tablespoons finely chopped fresh chives
2 tablespoons finely chopped fresh tarragon
4 tablespoons vinaigrette dressing (page 89)
150 g hard goat's cheese, feta cheese or mozzarella

In a bowl, put the escarole, radishes, olives, anchovies, tomatoes, shallot, chives and tarragon. Add the vinaigrette, toss gently and sprinkle over the cheese. Refrigerate for 30 minutes before serving.

pineapple and cucumber salad

300 g cucumber, peeled and thinly sliced
Salt
300 g fresh pineapple, diced
2 tablespoons light mayonnaise or single cream mixed with lemon juice (optional)
A few borage leaves in vinegar (page 116), fresh borage flowers or mint leaves

Put the cucumber into a colander, sprinkle with salt to extract the juice and leave for 45 minutes. Rinse away the salt and squeeze the water from the cucumber. In a bowl, mix the cucumber slices and diced pineapple and refrigerate for 2 hours. Before serving, drain away any excess water, toss in the mayonnaise or cream if using and decorate with the borage or mint.

warm asparagus salad

1 kg fresh thick asparagus, trimmed (remove woody ends)
Salt and pepper
6 tablespoons olive oil
2 tablespoons finely chopped fresh chervil (optional)
A few capers
Parmesan cheese shavings
Balsamic vinegar

In a roasting tin, place the asparagus in a single layer (avoid overcrowding) and season well. Pour over the olive oil and roast in a preheated oven at 200°C/gas mark 6 for about 20 minutes or until tender. Carefully place the cooked asparagus on a warm serving dish and sprinkle with the chervil (if using) capers, Parmesan cheese and a little balsamic vinegar. Serve warm.

parsley, onion and lemon salad

Serve as a side dish with grilled fish.

2 tablespoons olive oil
1 bunch parsley or chervil, finely chopped
1 large red onion, thinly sliced
2 lemons, peeled and diced
Salt and pepper
To serve: lettuce leaves

Mix all the ingredients in a bowl. Chill before serving. Serve on a bed of lettuce leaves.

black radish salad

1 or 2 black radish (depending on size), peeled and sliced
Salt (to sprinkle on radish)
150 g Gruyere or a cheese of your choice, finely diced
3 tablespoons vinaigrette dressing (page 89)
2 tablespoons finely chopped fresh parsley
1 shallot, finely chopped
1 lettuce

Put the radish in a colander, sprinkle with salt to extract the juice and leave for 45 minutes. Rinse the salt off and press down gently on the radish to squeeze out excess water. Mix the radish with some chunks of cheese in a salad bowl and add the vinaigrette. Sprinkle over the parsley and shallot, and lightly toss all the ingredients. Serve on a bed of lettuce.

cucumber salad

1 large cucumber, peeled and thinly sliced
Salt (to sprinkle on cucumber)
2 tablespoons finely chopped fresh chervil or flat-leaf parsley
1 shallot, finely chopped
100 g cooked ham or turkey, diced
4 tablespoons vinaigrette dressing (page 89)
Salt and pepper

Put the cucumber into a colander, sprinkle with salt to extract the juice and leave for 45 minutes. Rinse the salt off and, in a bowl, mix with the chervil or flat-leaf parsley, shallot and cooked ham or turkey. Toss in vinaigrette, add salt and pepper to taste and refrigerate before serving.

starters. main courses and accompaniments

The following recipes serve 4 people unless otherwise stated. Where possible, harvest your own ingredients or use fresh, organic produce. Take care to wash ingredients thoroughly.

STARTERS

taboule *(below)*

This dish can be served as a starter or a main course. To serve as a main course, double the amount of bulgar wheat in the recipe and add olives, preserved lemon slices (page 39), diced cucumber and a few chopped hard-boiled eggs.

120 g bulgar wheat (or couscous)
Salt and pepper
10 tablespoons olive oil
Juice of 1 lemon
300 g parsley, finely chopped
100 g mint, finely chopped
3 medium shallots or spring onions, chopped
To serve: ½ lettuce and 2 tomatoes, diced

Soak the bulgar wheat or couscous in warm water for about 15 minutes (or as indicated on the packet). In a sieve, drain well, pressing the grains to remove any excess water. Put the bulgar wheat or couscous in a bowl and add the salt, pepper, olive oil and lemon juice. Allow the wheat to absorb the dressing, then add the parsley, mint and shallots or spring onions. Refrigerate for 24 hours and then serve on a bed of lettuce garnished with the tomatoes.

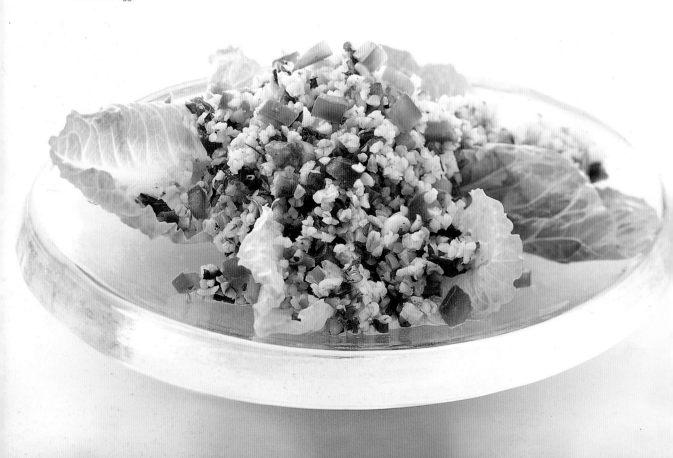

roman-style artichoke

This dish is excellent served cold a day after making.

50 g parsley, finely chopped
1 tablespoon finely chopped mint leaves
1 clove of garlic, crushed
Salt and pepper
2 tablespoons olive oil
4 medium or 8 small globe artichokes
Juice of half a lemon
250 ml olive oil

Mix the parsley and mint with the garlic, salt, pepper and 2 tablespoons of olive oil. Rinse the artichokes in water. Remove the outer, damaged leaves and the middle leaves. Trim the stalks off each choke (the centre) and remove the chokes using a curved, serrated grapefruit knife. Spoon the herb mixture into the middle of each artichoke and press the remaining leaves around the mixture. In a large casserole dish, cover the artichokes with salted water and 250 ml of olive oil. Bring slowly to the boil, then transfer the casserole dish to an oven preheated to 180°C/gas mark 4 for about 35 minutes or until cooked. Serve hot.

avocado tartar *(right)*

This can be served as a dip with carrot sticks or on toast.

2 avocados, peeled and stoned
2 shallots, finely chopped
1 tablespoon finely chopped tarragon
1 tablespoon finely chopped chervil
Juice of half a lemon
Salt and pepper

Put the ingredients in a blender and whizz. Refrigerate before serving.

cottage cheese with watercress

Serve as a starter, or as a snack on toast.

1 bunch watercress
1 tablespoon vinegar
250 g low-fat cottage cheese
Salt and pepper
1 tablespoon finely chopped parsley and shallots (optional)

Wash the watercress in a bowl of cold water with the vinegar. Dry the watercress, chop finely and combine with the cottage cheese. Season with salt and pepper and a mixture of the parsley and shallots, if desired.

green olive tapenade

Serve on toast, with eggs or as a sauce for pasta.

1 clove of garlic, peeled
1 tablespoon finely chopped tarragon
1 tablespoon finely chopped parsley
1 or 2 anchovies, soaked in milk for 10 minutes
3 tablespoons olive oil
Juice of half a small lemon
100 g small green olives, stoned and finely chopped
Salt and pepper

In a food processor blend the garlic, tarragon, parsley, anchovies, olive oil and lemon juice. Add the olives to the herb and oil mixture and season with salt and pepper.

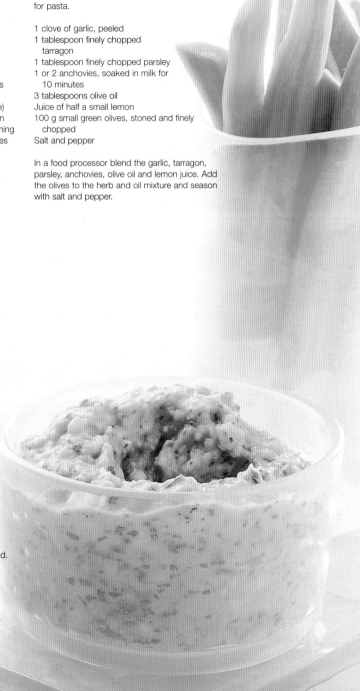

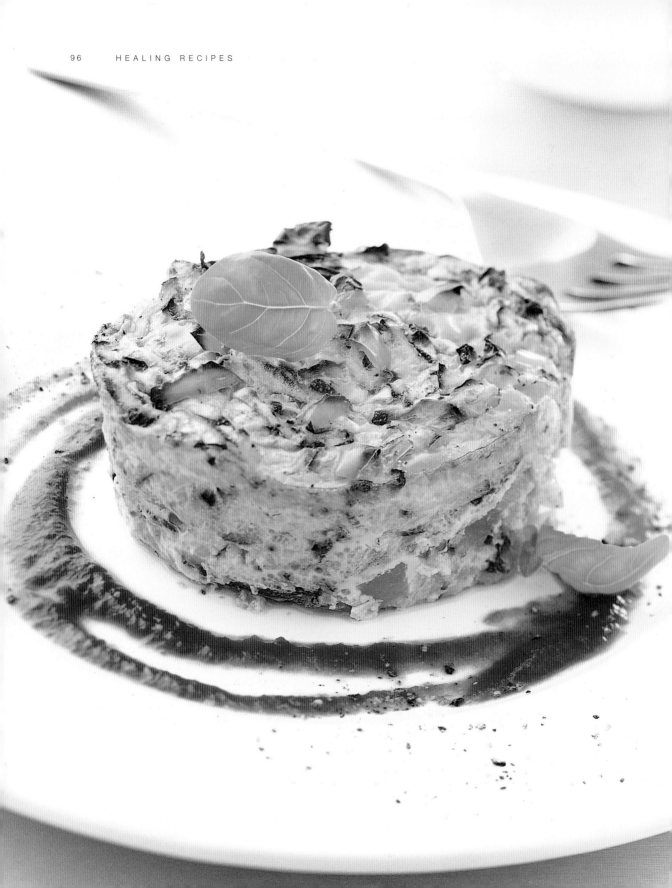

courgette cake *(left)*

800 g courgettes, roughly chopped
1 egg
3 tablespoons cottage cheese or ricotta cheese
Salt and pepper
1 yellow pepper, finely diced
To serve: tomato coulis (see below)

Boil the courgettes for approximately 4 minutes. In a food processor, blend them with the egg, cottage cheese or ricotta, and salt and pepper. Stir in the diced pepper. Divide the mixture between 4 individual dishes and place in a roasting tin, half-filled with hot water. Bake in a preheated oven at 170ºC/gas mark 3 for 25 minutes. Serve hot with tomato coulis.

tomato coulis

Serve with courgette cake (see previous recipe).

4 ripe beef tomatoes, quartered
Pinch of sugar
1 teaspoon tomato purée
4 tablespoons olive oil
Salt and pepper

In a food processor, blend the ingredients to an emulsion. Sieve to remove skin and seeds and use as required. Serve as a starter or as an accompaniment to grilled meat.

MAIN COURSES
nettle risotto

See page 88 for instructions on harvesting nettles. If nettles are out of season, use young spinach leaves instead.

2 medium onions, sliced
2 tablespoons olive oil
400 g risotto rice
150 ml dry white wine
1 litre vegetable or chicken stock, kept hot
200 g nettle tops
Salt and pepper
115 g Parmesan cheese, freshly grated
2 tablespoons finely chopped chervil or parsley

In a heavy-based saucepan, gently sweat the onions in the olive oil for about 10 minutes. Stir in the rice to coat with oil and cook for about 2 minutes. Pour in the wine and cook until the rice has absorbed all the liquid. Add the vegetable or chicken stock, a ladleful at a time, allowing the rice to absorb it all before adding more. Continue until the rice is cooked, but still retaining bite – the risotto should be loose and creamy. Meanwhile, steam the nettles until thoroughly wilted. Squeeze lightly and chop roughly. Stir into the risotto and heat through for 2 minutes. Season well and serve immediately, sprinkled with Parmesan and chervil or parsley.

buckwheat with leek sauce

Buckwheat comes either green or roasted. Green buckwheat has a much improved flavour if it is dry-roasted first. Cook it on its own in a pan, stirring all the time until there is a nutty, toasted aroma.

500 g dry-roasted green buckwheat
1 litre water
4 large leeks, chopped
3 eggs, beaten
Salt and pepper

For the sauce:
Half the cooked leeks (see recipe)
150 ml single cream, soya milk, cottage cheese or yoghurt
3 tablespoons chopped chervil or parsley
Lemon juice to taste

In a wide, heavy-based saucepan, bring the dry-roasted buckwheat and water to the boil. Simmer, covered, for 15–20 minutes or until the buckwheat is cooked. The buckwheat will absorb all the liquid and be light and fluffy in texture. Steam the leeks for 10 minutes or until cooked and divide in half. Combine one half of the leeks with the buckwheat and eggs. Season well and pour into a greased, ovenproof dish. Bake in a preheated oven at 180ºC/gas mark 4 for 20 minutes or until browned. Meanwhile, blend the remaining half of the leeks with the cream, soya milk, cottage cheese or yoghurt, and the chervil or parsley. Add lemon juice to taste. Re-heat (carefully if using single cream or yoghurt) and serve with the baked buckwheat and leek.

grilled salmon with aubergine sauce

3 large aubergines
6 tablespoons olive oil
Salt and pepper
2 tablespoons finely chopped basil
4 salmon fillets

Using a fork, prick the aubergines all over and cook under a preheated grill, set to maximum, turning them until the skins are completely charred. When cool enough to handle, peel. Put into a sieve and, using a saucer or a small plate, press out as much juice as possible. Pound the flesh in a mortar and slowly beat in the olive oil as if making mayonnaise. Alternatively, use a food processor and drizzle oil through the feeder. Season with salt and pepper. Add the basil. Under a preheated grill set to maximum, grill the salmon for 5 minutes on either side. Serve with a dollop of the aubergine sauce.

stuffed peppers *(below)*

225 ml salted water
115 g basmati rice, rinsed
2 green peppers
2 red peppers
1 large tomato, chopped
1 tablespoon chopped tarragon
100 g green and/or black olives, stoned and chopped
1 clove of garlic, crushed
1 teaspoon oil or butter
Salt and pepper

In a medium saucepan, bring the salted water to the boil. Add the rice and cook, covered, over a low heat for about 20 minutes or until the water is fully absorbed. Slice the tops off the peppers, remove the core and seeds and set aside. Stir the remaining ingredients into the cooked rice. Fill the peppers with the rice mixture and replace the tops. Put into an oiled, ovenproof dish and cover. Bake in a preheated oven at 180°C/gas mark 4 for about 35–40 minutes or until cooked.

buckwheat pancakes with field mushrooms

For the stuffing:
2 tablespoons vegetable oil
1 large onion, finely chopped
2 large cloves of garlic, crushed
1 teaspoon paprika
675 g field mushrooms, cut into 1-cm chunks
1 red pepper, seeded and cut into 1-cm chunks
150 ml red wine
4 large sage leaves, roughly chopped
3 tablespoons finely chopped parsley
Salt and pepper

For the pancakes:
225 g buckwheat flour
1 teaspoon salt
1 large egg
½ litre water
Oil to fry

In a large frying pan, heat the oil and cook the onion and garlic over a low heat for about 10 minutes or until soft. Add the paprika and mushroom chunks and stir. Add the pepper chunks and wine and cook for a further 10 minutes until all the moisture has evaporated. Stir through the herbs and season. Keep warm while you make the pancakes. To make the batter, put the flour and salt into a large bowl and make a well in the middle. Put the egg into the well and beat together. Gradually add the water. Refrigerate for at least 30 minutes, overnight if desired. Pour a small ladleful of batter into a hot, lightly oiled frying pan and cook on each side over a moderate heat for about 3–4 minutes or until lightly browned. Stack on a plate and keep warm. Place a little mushroom stuffing in the middle of each pancake, roll up and serve.

pasta twists with pesto

For the pesto:
5 cloves of garlic
15 large basil leaves (more for a stronger flavour)
50 g pine nuts
Salt and pepper
100 g Parmesan cheese, grated
100 ml olive oil

500 g fusilli pasta twists

Using a pestle and mortar, crush the garlic, basil and pine nuts (or use a blender). Add the salt, pepper, Parmesan and olive oil to make an emulsion. Bring a large pan of salted water to the boil. Add the pasta and return to the boil. Cook uncovered for about 12 minutes or until al dente. Do not drain the pasta completely as a little cooking water will help the pesto to coat the pasta. Toss generously in pesto and serve immediately.

leek and chive mimosa with polenta

4 leeks, coarse outer leaves removed
4 eggs, hard-boiled
2 tablespoons olive oil
2 tablespoons chopped chives, chervil, parsley or tarragon
4 lemon wedges

For the polenta:
250 g instant polenta
200 ml soya cream
1–2 tablespoons hot chilli sauce, or to taste
200 g Parmesan cheese or a strong cheddar, grated
Salt and pepper

Cut the leeks lengthways, rinse well under cold, running water and then boil in salted water (or steam) until tender. While the leeks are cooking, separate the yolks and the whites of the eggs, and mash separately with a fork. Boil the polenta according to the instructions on the packet and then stir through the cream, chilli sauce and cheese. Season well. To assemble: spoon the polenta onto a warmed serving dish and arrange the leeks on top. Sprinkle over the mashed egg whites and yolks. Keep warm. In a small frying pan, heat the olive oil, add the chives or other herbs, fry for about 30 seconds and pour over the leeks. Serve immediately with the lemon wedges.

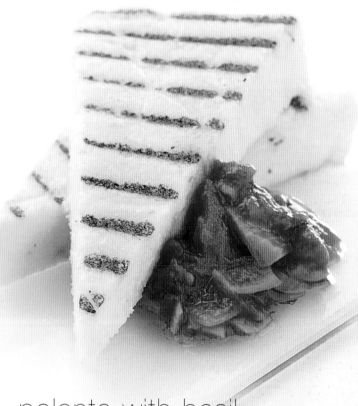

lamb with spinach and lentils

As a vegetarian alternative, the spinach and lentil mixture can be served with boiled rice instead of lamb.

225 g brown lentils, soaked overnight
1 large clove of garlic
500 g fresh spinach, cut into thin strips
1 tablespoon vegetable oil
½ teaspoon ground coriander
½ teaspoon ground cumin
Salt and pepper
4 tablespoons olive oil
2 tablespoons finely chopped coriander leaves
2 tablespoons plain yoghurt (optional)
2 lamb fillets, trimmed
Oil to fry

In a large saucepan of boiling water, cook the lentils with the garlic for about 15 minutes or until soft but not mushy. Pan-fry the spinach quickly in the vegetable oil until all excess moisture has evaporated. Add the spinach, coriander, cumin, seasoning and olive oil to the lentils. Just before serving, stir through the coriander and plain yoghurt, if using. In a very hot frying pan, fry the lamb fillets quickly on all sides, turning them over with a wooden spoon, for about 12 minutes or until they are well browned and crisp on the outside. (For well-done fillets, cook on the top shelf of a preheated oven at 230ºC/gas mark 8 for a further 10 minutes.) Slice the fillets thickly and serve on a bed of the spinach and lentil mixture.

polenta with basil tomato sauce *(above)*

For the sauce:
1 medium onion, chopped
2 tablespoons olive oil
500 g tomatoes
Handful of basil leaves, chopped
Salt and pepper

For the polenta:
1½ litres water
1 teaspoon salt
375 g pre-cooked polenta
100 g butter
200 g Parmesan cheese, grated

Using a heavy-based saucepan, gently sweat the onion in the olive oil over a low heat. Peel the tomatoes (plunging them in boiling water helps the skin to come away) and add to the onions. Season and simmer for 30–40 minutes. When the sauce is thick and pulpy, add the basil and remove from the heat. Using a heavy-based saucepan, bring the water and salt to the boil, stir in the polenta and cook over a low heat for about 10 minutes, stirring all the time. Stir in the butter and Parmesan cheese and transfer to a rectangular, shallow dish. Spread level with a spatula and allow to set solid. Cut into slices, reheat in the oven or microwave, or by grilling, and serve with a generous portion of basil tomato sauce.

chicken breasts with celeriac mash *(below)*

4 skinless chicken breasts
Pepper
4 lettuce, large spinach or sorrel leaves
8 slices smoked streaky bacon
Oil to fry

For the mash:
1 celeriac, peeled and cut into chunks
Same weight of potatoes, peeled and cut into chunks
A little hot milk
Olive oil or butter to taste
Salt and pepper

Make a slit the length of the chicken breasts and open like a book. Grind pepper into the opening and cover with a lettuce, spinach or sorrel leaf. Close up the breasts and wrap each one in two pieces of bacon. Secure with a toothpick. Refrigerate until ready to use. In two large saucepans, boil the celeriac and potatoes separately until cooked. Drain and transfer into one large pan. Cover with a clean folded tea towel to absorb any steam. Mash the vegetables together, beat in a little hot milk, olive oil or butter to make a creamy consistency and season to taste. Keep warm. In a frying pan, heat the oil and cook the chicken breasts for about 12 minutes or until they are brown on all sides and the juices run clear. Serve with the celeriac mash.

dandelion, bacon and potato cakes

Pancetta or smoked ham can be used instead of bacon. If using smoked ham, add just before serving. Dandelion, bacon and potato cakes are delicious served with green bean salad (page 91).

115 g smoked, streaky bacon, chopped and rind removed
1 tablespoon vegetable oil
500 g young dandelion leaves (or destalked watercress, or lettuce)
2 cloves of garlic
2 tablespoons white wine vinegar
500 g potatoes, boiled and mashed
2 tablespoons flour
1 large egg
Oil to fry

In a large, heavy-based frying pan, fry the bacon in the oil. When cooked, remove and set aside. Add the dandelion leaves, watercress or lettuce and the garlic to the pan. Soften over a low heat for about 12 minutes or until cooked. Remove the garlic, add the vinegar and continue cooking until the liquid has evaporated and the mixture is quite dry. Mix the leaf mixture into the mashed potato together with the bacon. Beat in the flour and egg thoroughly. With floured hands, make into 4 large or 8 small equal patties and fry in hot oil until they are golden brown on both sides. Serve piping hot.

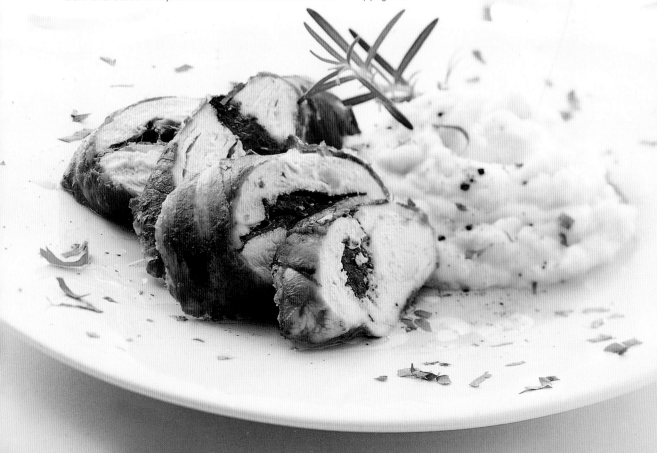

baked pumpkin strudel

3 tablespoons olive oil
2 red onions, finely chopped
800 g pumpkin or squash flesh, cut into small chunks
2 cloves of garlic, crushed
1 bay leaf
Sprig of fresh thyme
Salt and pepper
1 x 400 g packet fresh filo pastry
Plenty of olive oil to brush
1 egg, beaten
115 g Parmesan cheese, freshly grated
55 g wholemeal breadcrumbs

In a 25-cm wide pan, heat the oil, add the onion and cook for 10 minutes or until soft. Add the pumpkin or squash, garlic, bay leaf, thyme and seasoning. Cover and cook over a low heat, allowing the ingredients to cook gently in their own juices. If the pumpkin starts to stick, stir in a little water. Allow to cool slightly. Lay out 4 overlapping sheets of filo pastry and brush quickly with oil. Cover with another 4 sheets and brush with oil. Repeat once more to make three layers. Spoon over the pumpkin mixture to within 5 cm of the edges and roll up into a sausage. Tuck the ends under. Slip a baking sheet underneath, brush with beaten egg and sprinkle over a mixture of Parmesan and breadcrumbs. Bake in a preheated oven at 200ºC/gas mark 6 for about 20 minutes or until the pastry and breadcrumb mixture is golden brown. Serve immediately.

chicken, millet, barley and celeriac pilaff

To make a seafood pilaff use a mixture of prawns, squid and mussels instead of chicken

4 chicken breasts, skinned
8 tablespoons olive oil
1 large clove of garlic, crushed
Salt and pepper
200 g millet
500 g celeriac, peeled and finely diced
200 g barley, soaked overnight
150 ml pesto (page 98)
Pepper
To serve: 8 large basil leaves

Marinate the chicken in the oil, garlic and seasoning for at least 2 hours. Cook the millet in twice its own volume of boiling water for about 10 minutes or until al dente. Meanwhile, steam the celeriac with the barley for 15 minutes or until both are cooked. Combine the celeriac, millet and barley, with plenty of pesto and pepper. Keep warm. In a frying pan, cook the chicken with the marinade juices for about 6 minutes on each side. When cool enough to handle, tear into strips and fork through the millet mixture. Tear the basil leaves and sprinkle over the top.

spicy spinach, prunes and beans

Cinnamon, chopped almonds, raisins and chopped parsley can be added to the couscous if desired. Alternatively, basmati rice can be used instead of couscous.

1 tablespoon oil
1 red onion, chopped
125 g black-eye beans (or other beans) soaked overnight
½ teaspoon ground turmeric
1 teaspoon ground cinnamon
Pepper
350 ml water
125 g no-soak prunes
1 kg young spinach leaves, picked over
225 g couscous

In a large saucepan, heat the oil and sweat the onion over a low heat for 10 minutes or until soft. Drain the beans and add to the pan along with the turmeric, cinnamon and pepper. Cover with the water and simmer with the lid on. When the beans are three-quarters cooked (probably after about 30 minutes), add the prunes. Add the spinach, in batches, to the stew and cook for a further 10 minutes. Cook the couscous according to the instructions on the packet and serve with the stew.

halibut steak and nettle butter

If nettles are out of season, use fresh sorrel leaves.

150 g young nettle leaves
150 g unsalted butter, softened
Salt and pepper
4 tablespoons white wine
4 tablespoons salted water or fish stock
1 bay leaf
Juice of half lemon
4 halibut steaks

Steam the nettles for about 8 minutes or until wilted. Squeeze dry. Blend the nettles and butter in a food processor and season to taste. Spread onto greaseproof paper and roll into a log. Refrigerate. Cut into discs when hard. In a large shallow pan bring the wine and salted water or fish stock to the boil, add the bay leaf and lemon juice. Add the halibut and simmer for 5 minutes on each side. Serve with black pepper and a disc of butter.

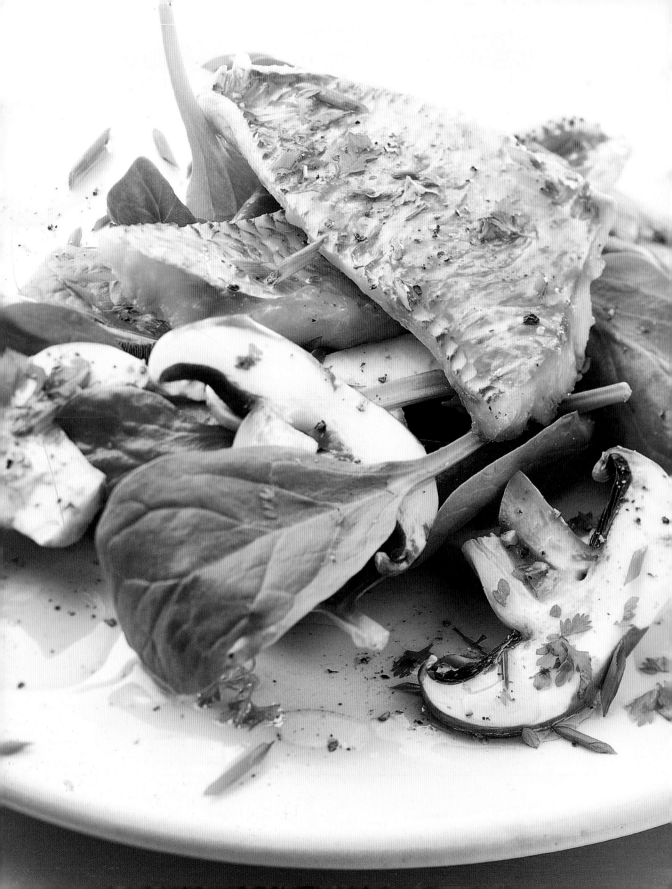

red mullet with raw spinach salad *(left)*

1.5 kg young spinach leaves, picked over
6 medium mushrooms, sliced
A few rocket leaves (optional)
Salt and pepper
3 tablespoons vinaigrette (page 89)
3 tablespoons oil
8 red mullet fillets
To serve: chervil and chives, chopped

Remove the stems from the spinach, place the leaves in a serving dish and add the mushrooms, rocket, salt and pepper. Toss in the vinaigrette. In a frying pan, heat the oil and rapidly sauté the mullet for 5 minutes on each side or until cooked. Place the mullet on the salad. Garnish with the chervil and chives.

ACCOMPANIMENTS

onions in cider *(below right)*

4 tablespoons oil
10 medium onions
25 ml dry cider
1 sprig rosemary
2 bay leaves
Salt and pepper
To serve: cooked courgettes

In a large frying pan, heat the oil and slowly fry the whole onions until they are golden brown all over. Add the cider, rosemary, bay leaves, salt and pepper, then cover and simmer gently until the onions are well cooked (they should retain their shape). Remove the onions and reduce the sauce by boiling rapidly to a syrupy consistency. Cover the onions with the sauce and serve with the courgettes.

steamed shallots

Serve as a main dish accompaniment or use to thicken sauces.

300 g shallots, peeled
½ teaspoon ground cinnamon

Steam the shallots, then blend in a food processor with the cinnamon.

rice with cucumber balls

500 ml salted water
250 g brown rice, rinsed
1 cucumber
1 shallot, finely chopped
30 g butter
1 tablespoon finely chopped coriander or parsley

In a large saucepan, bring the salted water to the boil. Add the rice and cook, covered, over a low heat for 20 minutes or until ready. Cut the cucumber in half lengthways and, using a melon baller, make as many balls as possible. Blanch the balls in boiling water for 2 minutes, then drain and rinse in cold water. In a frying pan, cook the shallot and cucumber in the butter over a low heat. As soon as they start to colour, add the rice and serve sprinkled with the coriander or parsley.

potato and watercress mash

500 g potatoes, peeled and chopped
300 g watercress, damaged stalks removed
1 tablespoon butter or single cream
Large pinch of nutmeg
Salt and pepper

Cook the potatoes in boiling, salted water. Drain and return to a low heat to drive off excess moisture. In a food processor, blend the watercress with the butter or cream. Add to the potato, and use a masher to make a smooth pureé. Stir in the nutmeg and salt and pepper.

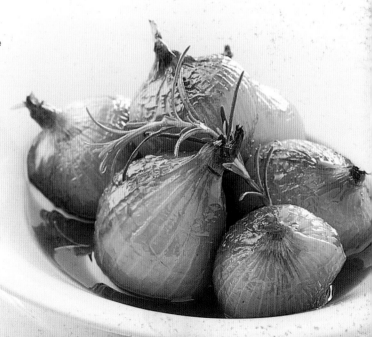

celery with wine and herbs

1 large head of celery (or 2 small ones)
75 ml white wine
75 ml water
4 tablespoons olive oil
2 tablespoons finely chopped parsley
2 tablespoons finely chopped tarragon
Salt and pepper
Lemon juice

Carefully wash the celery and remove the root, leaves and stringy parts of the stalks. Cut into small pieces and cook in boiling, salted water for 4–6 minutes. Drain (the cooking water can be kept and used in a soup) and place in an ovenproof dish. Boil the wine and water for 1 minute, then pour over the celery in the ovenproof dish. Add the olive oil and cook for 20 minutes at 170ºC/gas mark 3. Add the parsley, tarragon and seasoning. Serve hot with a few drops of lemon juice.

peas with bacon pieces

100 g lardons or chopped lean bacon, rind removed
500 g fresh or frozen peas or 500 g can pease pudding
150 ml vegetable stock
Rocket, finely chopped
Black pepper

In a frying pan, sauté the lardons or bacon until golden. Drain away the fat and set aside. In a food processor, blend the peas, if using, with the vegetable stock. Transfer the pea mixture or pease pudding to the frying pan and heat. Mix the lardons or bacon with the pea mixture or pease pudding. Transfer to a serving dish. Sprinkle over the rocket and pepper.

salsify

Salsify will keep well in the refrigerator for a few days and is an interesting accompaniment to main courses. Canned salsify can be used instead of fresh; just sauté before serving.

1½ litres cold water
1 tablespoon plain flour
3 tablespoons vinegar
10 g salt
1 kg fresh salsify
Olive oil
1 tablespoon finely chopped parsley

In a large pan, mix the water, flour, vinegar and salt. Bring to the boil, stirring well. Plunge the salsify into the boiling water, then cover and simmer for 20 minutes or until cooked. (Cool and store the salsify in its cooking water in the refrigerator.) Before serving, lightly sauté in olive oil and garnish with the parsley.

brussels sprouts with chestnuts

600 g chestnuts
1 litre meat or vegetable stock
750 g Brussels sprouts, damaged outer leaves removed
100 g chopped bacon, lardons or pancetta, rind removed
1 tablespoon vegetable oil

Using a sharp knife, make an incision in each chestnut. Place the chestnuts in a pan and cover with cold water. Bring to the boil for 2 minutes, drain and peel the outer and inner skin. Cook the peeled chestnuts in the meat or vegetable stock for 30 minutes. Cook the Brussels sprouts for about 15 minutes in salted, boiling water (the sprouts should remain firm). Using a frying pan, sauté the bacon, lardons or pancetta in the oil. When cooked, drain the fat and add the sprouts and chestnuts to the pan. Mix by shaking the pan, heat through for 4 minutes. Season to taste and serve immediately.

beans with carrots and onions

This is an excellent accompaniment to sausages or red meat.

200 g onions, sliced
200 g carrots, diced
3 cloves of garlic
150 ml olive oil or 30 g butter
1 kg dried beans (flageolet, red kidney or borlotti beans), soaked overnight
Bouquet garni (made with a bay leaf, 2 or 3 sprigs of thyme, 2 or 3 sprigs of parsley and 1 clove)
Salt and pepper

In a large saucepan, cook the onions, carrots and garlic in the olive oil or butter over a low heat for approximately 10 minutes or until the onions are soft. Stir frequently. Add the drained beans and cook for 3 minutes, then cover with water and bring to the boil. Add the bouquet garni, cover and simmer for 1½ hours or until the beans are cooked. Add salt and pepper after 45 minutes. Serve hot.

fennel with wine

This dish goes very well with smoked fish or cold meat.

800 g fennel, bruised outer layer and tops removed
300 ml white wine
2 bay leaves
1 cinnamon stick or ½ teaspoon ground cinnamon
A few crushed black peppercorns
30 g pistachio nuts, shelled
2 anchovy fillets (optional)
1 teaspoon sugar
Pinch of nutmeg
3 tablespoons olive oil

1 tablespoon vinegar
Juice and grated zest of half a lemon

Cut the fennel into quarters and slice thinly. In a saucepan, put the white wine, bay leaves, cinnamon, peppercorns and fennel, and cover with water. Bring to the boil, then cover and simmer until the fennel is cooked but still firm. Strain the fennel and put into a deep dish. Blend the pistachio, anchovy (if using), sugar, nutmeg, olive oil, vinegar and lemon in a food processor and spoon the sauce over the fennel. Cover with cling film and refrigerate for 24 hours. Serve at room temperature.

potatoes with herb sauce

For the sauce:
Small bunch (5 or 6 sprigs) of parsley, finely chopped
Small bunch (5 or 6 sprigs) of chervil, finely chopped
2 tablespoons tarragon leaves, finely chopped
4 anchovy fillets (optional), finely chopped
1 egg, hard-boiled and finely chopped
2 small shallots, finely chopped
Pinch of black pepper
3 tablespoons olive oil
1 tablespoon white wine vinegar
1 tablespoon white wine

16 small new or salad potatoes, boiled
2 teaspoons fresh capers (replace with preserved capers if necessary)

Make the sauce by mixing the ingredients together (boil the white wine briefly before mixing, in order to allow the alcohol to evaporate). Slice the boiled potatoes while hot and place them in a serving dish. Warm the sauce over a gentle heat and then pour on the potatoes. Sprinkle over the capers and toss very gently. Serve warm.

green beans with dijon mustard (right)

1 kg green beans
150 g single cream or yoghurt
Juice of 1 small lemon
1 tablespoon Dijon mustard
100 g toasted, chopped hazelnuts
Salt and pepper

Using a steamer, cook the green beans until al dente. Rinse in cold water and then drain. Mix the cream or yoghurt, lemon juice and mustard in a bowl, then add the beans and toss lightly. Sprinkle over the toasted hazelnuts, season and refrigerate before serving.

cardamom hot sauce

Use this sauce to add flavour to soups or stews.

1 teaspoon black peppercorns
1 teaspoon caraway seeds
4 cardamom pods
4 dried chillies
1 bulb of garlic, peeled
Bunch of coriander leaves, washed with stems removed

In a food processor, blend all of the ingredients and use as desired.

horseradish sauce

Adjust the ingredients according to taste. Use as a condiment.

20 g shallots, finely chopped
Pinch of ground black pepper
50 g salt
200 g mustard powder
1 dried red chilli, ground
60 g fresh horseradish root, grated
1 teaspoon grated nutmeg
125 ml vinegar
50 ml dry white wine
A little vegetable stock

In a food processor, blend all the ingredients into a smooth paste. If the mixture is too dry, add some vegetable stock. To reduce the strength and sharpness, boil the blended ingredients for 5 minutes. Refrigerate.

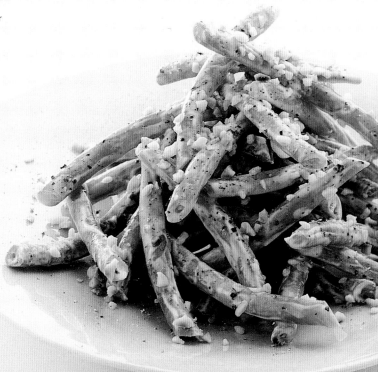

desserts

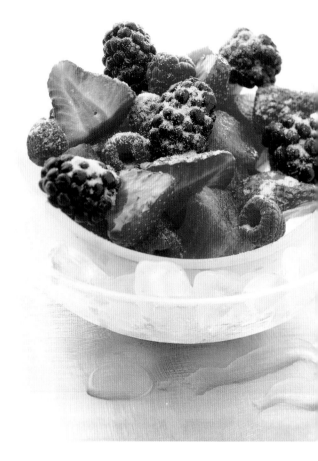

The following recipes serve 4 people unless otherwise stated. Where possible, harvest your own ingredients or use fresh, organic produce. Take care to wash thoroughly, peel or de-seed fruit where necessary.

watermelon and summer fruits *(right)*

1 small watermelon
Blackberries (frozen if out of season)*
Raspberries*
Strawberries*
Crushed ice
Caster sugar to taste
2 tablespoons orange-blossom water (available in health shops and
   supermarkets)

* Use one quarter of the weight of the watermelon of each fruit.

Cut off the top of the watermelon and spoon out all the flesh. Remove the seeds and cut the flesh into rough cubes. Mix with the other fruit and a small amount of crushed ice. Use this fruit mixture to fill up the shell of the watermelon. Sprinkle on caster sugar and orange-blossom water. Alternatively, serve the fruit salad in individual bowls.

banana and date salad

5 ripe bananas, peeled and sliced
250 g fresh dates, stoned and finely chopped
300 ml live yoghurt
To decorate: toasted chopped nuts

In glass bowls, arrange the bananas and dates in alternate layers and pour on the yoghurt. Refrigerate overnight. Serve sprinkled with toasted chopped nuts if desired.

lychee fruit salad

200 g lychees, peeled and stoned
200 g tangerines, peeled and separated into segments
6–8 kumquats, chopped
2 tablespoons orange-blossom water
2 glasses crushed ice made with jasmine tea

Put the fruit in a bowl and pour over the orange-blossom water and crushed ice. Serve immediately.

minted melon

2 tablespoons granulated sugar
2 tablespoons water
3 tablespoons fresh mint leaves
Juice of half a lemon
1 ripe honeydew melon, refrigerated
A few chunks crystallized ginger or ginger preserved in syrup (optional)

In a small saucepan, over a low heat, completely dissolve the sugar in the water. Bring to the boil and add the mint and lemon juice. Cool. Slice the melon and place in glass bowls. Glaze the melon with the cold syrup. Serve with ginger if desired.

pumpkin in syrup

1 medium pumpkin
750 g sugar
½ litre water
To decorate: walnuts and toasted almonds, chopped

Cut the pumpkin into eight wedges, cut the flesh from the peel and remove the seeds and fibres. Dissolve the sugar completely in the water. Bring to the boil and add the pumpkin wedges. Simmer for 20 minutes or until tender: the bubbles should become bigger and slower. Allow to cool and serve the pumpkin and syrup sprinkled with the walnuts and toasted almonds.

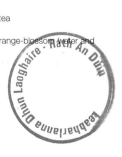

rhubarb and ginger tart

For the shortcrust pastry:
225 g plain flour
Pinch of salt
110 g butter
3 tablespoons ice-cold water

For the filling:
500 g fresh rhubarb stalks, washed
100 g soft brown sugar
5-cm piece root ginger, peeled and grated, or 1 teaspoon orange or
   lemon zest
1 tablespoon lemon juice
To serve: fresh cream or live yoghurt (optional)

To make the shortcrust pastry: blend the flour, salt and butter in a food processor until well combined. Mix in enough water to bind. Chill for 30 minutes and then use the pastry to line a 25-cm tart tin. Cut the rhubarb into small chunks (about 1.5 cm long). Stack the chunks tightly in the pastry case and sprinkle with the brown sugar, ginger and lemon juice. Bake immediately in an oven preheated to 180ºC/gas mark 4 for 35 minutes or until cooked. Serve with a little fresh cream or live yoghurt if desired.

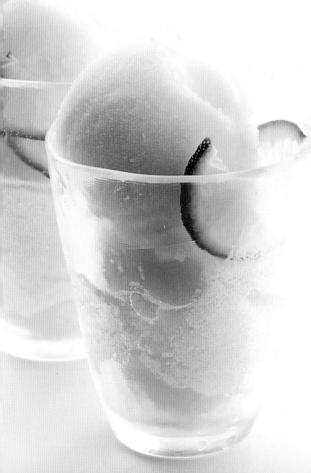

fruit salad with lemon balm

100 g wild strawberries
100 g blackberries
100 g blueberries
100 g redcurrants
3 dessert apples peeled, cored, sliced and sprinkled with lemon juice
100 g sugar
75 ml water
150 ml sparkling wine (optional)
2 tablespoons lemon juice
10 lemon-balm leaves, finely chopped

In a large bowl mix the fruit together. Over a low heat, dissolve the sugar in the water, wine (if using) and lemon juice. Bring to the boil and reduce to a syrup. When the syrup has cooled, pour it over the fruit and sprinkle the lemon-balm leaves on top. Refrigerate for at least 2 hours before serving.

red- and whitecurrants with raspberry coulis

250 g redcurrants
250 g whitecurrants
250 g raspberries
100 g sugar
To decorate: fresh mint leaves
To serve: fresh cream or live yoghurt (optional)

Combine the red- and whitecurrants and arrange in individual glass bowls. Crush the raspberries with a fork or blend in a food processor. Transfer to a stainless steel, enamel or glass pan and cook over a medium heat for 2 minutes. Strain through a fine sieve into a clean pan and, over a low heat, dissolve the sugar in the juice. Pour, warm, over the red and whitecurrants. Decorate with the mint. Serve with fresh cream or live yoghurt if desired.

fresh mint sorbet (left)

200 g sugar
300 ml water
3 tablespoons fresh mint leaves, washed and dried
Juice of 2 lemons
1 egg white
To decorate: whole mint leaves or lime slices (optional)

In a large saucepan, over a low heat, dissolve the sugar completely in the water. Bring to the boil and reduce until syrupy. Meanwhile, chop the mint finely (setting some aside for the decoration if desired), add to the cooling syrup and allow to infuse for 1 hour. Strain, stir in the lemon juice and freeze until set. Break the frozen syrup into pieces and blend in a food processor. Whisk the egg white until stiff and fold in. Decorate with whole mint leaves or lime slices if desired and serve.

pears with herbs

1 litre boiling water
1 handful lime flowers (linden)
2 tablespoons dried mint
2 star anise
Zest of 1 orange
4 large pears
Sugar to taste
Dried fruit such as apricots, sultanas or prunes (optional)
To decorate: toasted nuts (optional)

Pour the boiling water over the lime flowers, mint, star anise and orange zest, cover and infuse for 30 minutes. Strain the infusion and then pour it into a large steamer or pressure cooker. Steam the pears with the infusion until they are tender (in a pressure cooker this should take about 4–5 minutes). Remove the pears, reduce the infusion by half and add sugar to taste. Pour the infusion over the pears in a serving dish and allow to cool before serving. If desired, you can add some dried fruit such as apricots, sultanas or prunes to the infusion before you pour it over the pears. They will swell in the liquid and take up the fragrance of the herbs. You can also serve the pears decorated with a sprinkling of toasted nuts.

autumn fruit compote

1 kg dessert apples, peeled, cored and roughly chopped
1 kg pears, peeled, cored and roughly chopped
500 g black grapes, de-seeded
Juice and grated zest of 1 lemon or 1 tablespoon grated fresh ginger
1 clove
½ teaspoon ground cinnamon
Pinch of nutmeg
150 ml water
To serve: fresh cream or live yoghurt (optional)

In a heavy-based saucepan, place the apples, pears and grapes with the lemon juice and add the remaining ingredients. Simmer for 25 minutes, or until all the fruit is cooked. Empty the fruit into a glass bowl and allow to cool. Serve with fresh cream or live yoghurt if desired.

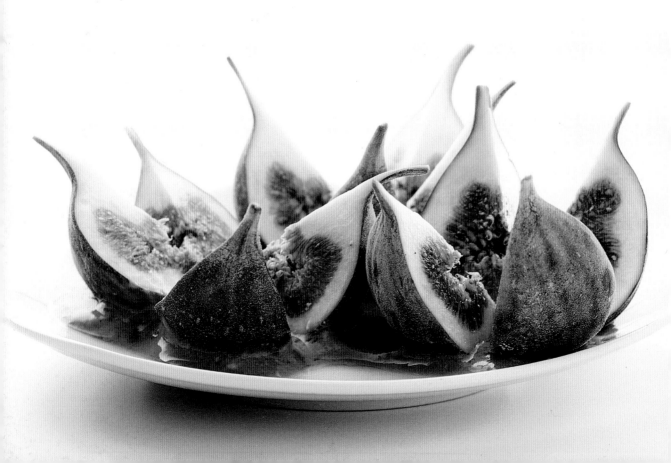

baked papaya with ginger

3 papayas, halved and de-seeded
60 g unsalted butter
5 chunks of preserved ginger, chopped
Juice and zest of 1 lime
1 tablespoon of preserved ginger syrup
To serve: brown sugar or honey to taste (optional)

Place the papayas in a buttered ovenproof dish. Mash together or blend the butter and ginger with half the lime juice and zest. Pour the mixture into the halved papayas. Sprinkle with the remaining lime juice, followed by the ginger syrup and brown sugar, if desired. Bake in the oven preheated to 180°C/gas mark 4 until tender, basting occasionally with the juices. Serve with a little honey spooned over the top if desired.

fresh figs with raspberry cheese *(left)*

12 figs
150 g raspberries
100 g cottage cheese
1 tablespoon caster sugar
3 tablespoons live yoghurt

Quarter the figs to within 1 cm of the base. In a food processor, blend the raspberries, then mix with the cottage cheese, sugar and yoghurt. Pour this mixture over the figs. Refrigerate for a few hours before serving.

poached apricots with cardamom *(right)*

4 cardamom pods
600 ml water
100 g brown or white sugar
Zest of 1 lemon, cut into thin strips
12 apricots, stoned
Orange juice to taste
To serve: toasted chopped nuts (optional)

Using a rolling pin, crush the cardamom pods and tie into a muslin bag. In a large saucepan, bring the water, sugar and lemon zest to the boil. Add the cardamom and simmer for a few minutes until the cardamom flavour is sufficiently strong (taste the syrup). Remove the muslin bag, add 12 apricots and poach for about 10 minutes over a low heat (the syrup should be barely simmering). Once the apricots are cooked, remove them and reduce the syrup by half by boiling rapidly. Add a little orange juice to taste and pour the syrup over the apricots. Serve chilled with toasted chopped nuts if desired.

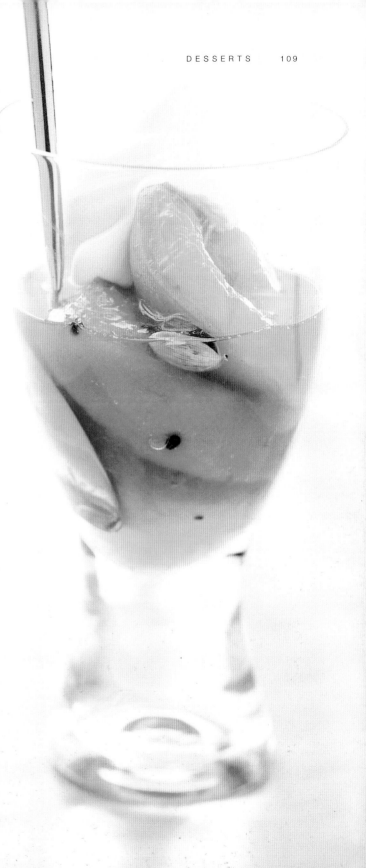

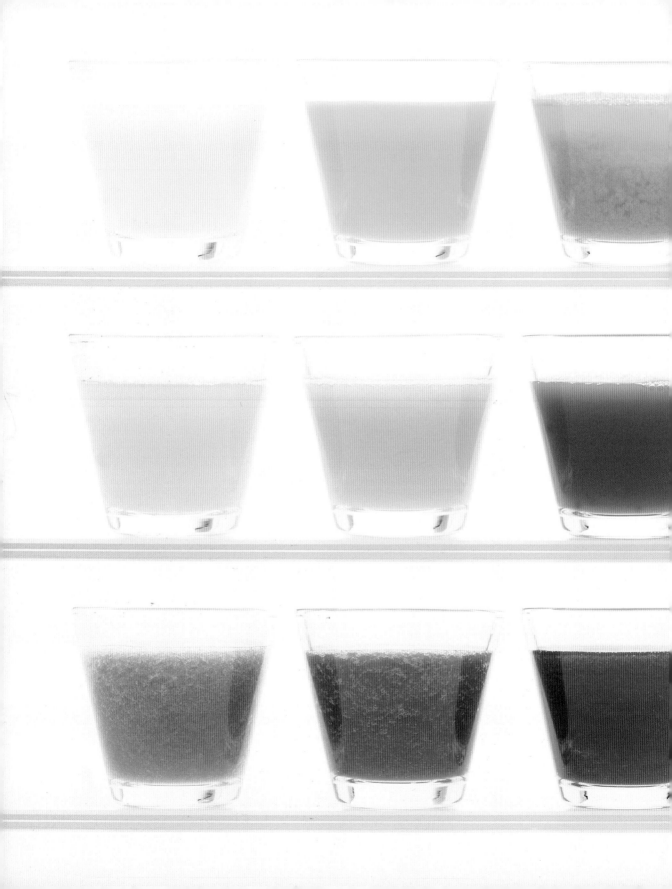

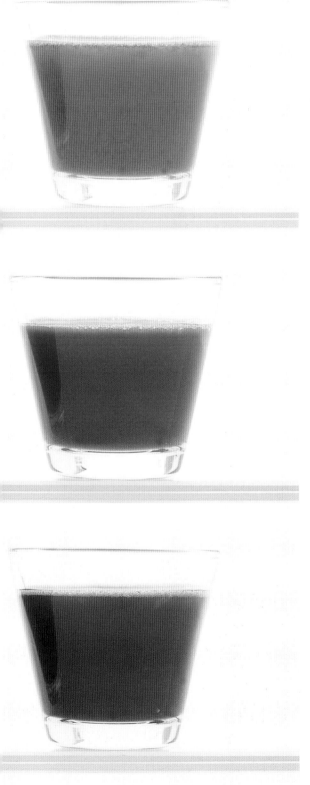

juices

To maximize the nutritional value of juice, use the freshest possible ingredients and drink the juice immediately (make a small quantity and drink it all at once rather than storing it). Where possible, harvest your own ingredients or use fresh, organic produce. Avoid using fruit and vegetables that are damaged or overripe and take care to wash ingredients thoroughly. If fruit is difficult to obtain, buy ready-made juice from a health-food shop – always choose brands that are organic and unsweetened.

The following juices are made using either a juicer or a blender. A juicer extracts the juice from fruit and vegetables, leaving behind the solid parts, such as the rind, peel, pith and pips – ideal for citrus fruit and apples. A blender simply liquidizes the whole fruit or vegetable – good for soft fruit such as strawberries and raspberries. If you do not have a juicer, you can add a little water to a recipe, blend the ingredients and then strain them through a sieve or a piece of muslin. Juices are best served cold, poured over crushed ice. Vegetable juices can be seasoned with salt and pepper.

Because is hard to predict how much juice individual fruits will yield, the amounts of fruit given in these recipes may need adjusting depending on water content (older, riper fruit yields more juice but may be less nutritious).

FRUIT JUICES

apple and raspberry juice

300 g dessert apples, peeled, cored and roughly chopped
100 g raspberries
2 tablespoons rosewater or orange-blossom water
Ice cubes made from jasmine tea
Sugar to taste

In a blender, blend the apples and raspberries. Add the rosewater or orange-blossom water, then pour the liquid over jasmine tea ice cubes. Alternatively, crush the jasmine tea ice cubes in the blender with the fruit. Add sugar to taste.

apricot, lime and mint juice

3 ripe apricots, stoned
3 tablespoons fresh lime juice
Honey to taste
1 teaspoon chopped fresh mint
Crushed ice

In a blender, blend the apricots and the lime juice. Sweeten to taste with honey and pour into a glass half-filled with mint and crushed ice.

cherry and raspberry juice

50 ml ready-made cherry juice
50 ml ready-made raspberry juice
Juice of half a lemon
Crushed ice

Mix the juices together and add the lemon juice and crushed ice.

cherry and apple juice

3 dessert apples
50 ml ready-made cherry juice

Process the apples in a juicer and mix the apple juice with the cherry juice.

mango juice

2 medium-sized mangoes, peeled and stoned
2 tablespoons orange-blossom water
A few ice cubes made from camomile tea

Using a blender, process the mango flesh with the orange-blossom water and the camomile ice cubes. Blend until the ice is well crushed.

carrot, apple and ginger juice

6 carrots, cut in chunks
4 apples, peeled, cored and cut in chunks
1 tablespoon grated root ginger
Crushed ice

Process the carrots, apples and ginger in a juicer. Pour over crushed ice.

prune juice

1 teaspoon lemon juice
Maple syrup to taste
150 ml ready-made prune juice

Mix the lemon juice and maple syrup with the prune juice.

redcurrant, blackberry and blueberry juice

100 g redcurrants
100 g blackberries
100 g blueberries

Use frozen fruits if redcurrants, blackberries or blueberries are out of season. Process the ingredients in a blender.

strawberry and raspberry juice

200 g strawberries
200 g raspberries
Lemon juice to taste
Crushed ice
A little water

In a blender, process the strawberries and raspberries. Add lemon juice and pour over crushed ice. Add water if necessary.

pineapple shake

100 ml soya milk
50 ml pineapple juice
1 teaspoon grated coconut
Sugar to taste

Using a blender, process the ingredients. Add sugar to taste. Serve chilled.

VEGETABLE JUICES

celery and tomato juice

Half a celery plant
2 tomatoes
1 cucumber

Trim the celery sticks and base. Process the ingredients in a juicer.

cabbage, carrot and celery juice

This juice can be served hot or cold.

½ red or white cabbage
4 carrots, roughly chopped
5 sticks celery, roughly chopped
½ red onion (or 2 shallots)
Water
Salt and pepper
1 teaspoon lemon juice

In a blender, blend the vegetables. Add a little water to thin the consistency and add salt, pepper and lemon juice.

green bean and garlic juice

230 g green beans
2 small lettuce hearts
2 tablespoons water
2 cloves of garlic
Pinch of cayenne pepper
Crushed ice

In a juicer, process the vegetables water and garlic, mix with the cayenne pepper and pour over the crushed ice.

black radish and carrot juice

100 g black radishes
50 g carrots

Process the ingredients in a juicer.

broccoli and green bean juice

A few stems and florets of broccoli
100 g green beans
2 tablespoons lemon juice
2 tablespoons water
Crushed ice

In a juicer, process the vegetables, mix with the water and pour over the crushed ice.

celery and red onion juice

1 celery plant, leaves and outside sticks removed
2 red onions
Crushed ice
Juice of half a lemon

Trim the celery sticks and base. In a juicer, process the celery and onions and pour over the crushed ice and lemon juice.

beetroot and celery juice

1 celery plant, leaves and outside sticks removed
2 medium-sized beetroots, cooked
Juice of half a lemon or lime
1 tablespoon olive oil

Trim the celery sticks and base. In a juicer, process the beetroots and celery and pour in a glass with the lemon juice and olive oil.

cucumber and lettuce heart juice

2 medium-sized cucumbers
1 lettuce heart

Process the ingredients in a juicer.

lettuce and basil juice

1 lettuce
1 radicchio
5 basil leaves
Juice of half a lemon

Process the lettuce, radicchio and basil in a juicer and then add the lemon juice.

pickles and preserves

When making preserves buy the best quality ingredients possible. Sterilize jars and bottles by pouring boiling water over them or leaving them in a hot oven for a few minutes. The main ingredient used in pickling is vinegar – this acts as a solvent, taking the aroma as well as the medicinally-active ingredients from the plants. Preserves should generally be consumed within three months.

PICKLED VEGETABLES

pickled turnips

Serve with main dishes, such as pork and potatoes.

1½ kg turnip, peeled and grated
30 g salt
40 juniper berries
30 black peppercorns

Place the ingredients in layers in a large glass or ceramic jar (do not use metal), then put a sterile cloth and a plate on the top layer. Place a weight on top of the plate and keep refrigerated. The turnips will start to ferment and will take 2–3 weeks to pickle. When pickled, rinse well in cold water and dry thoroughly. Serve raw in salad or cook and serve in the same way as sauerkraut (boiled and as an accompaniment for sausages or pork).

pickled beetroot

1 kg baby beetroot, unpeeled
1 litre water
½ litre red wine vinegar
2 bay leaves
2 sprigs of thyme
12 black peppercorns
2 cloves of garlic
50 g salt
100 g granulated sugar
1 white onion, sliced

Wrap the beetroot in foil and bake in a preheated oven at 200°C/gas mark 6 until tender. Meanwhile, bring the water, vinegar, herbs, peppercorns, garlic, salt and sugar to the boil and cook for 3 minutes. Leave to cool. Peel the beetroot and combine with the onion in hermetically-sealable pickling jars. Pour over the pickling vinegar and seal the jars tightly. Store for at least 2 weeks in a cool, dark place.

pickled cauliflower _(right)_

Use in starters or salads.

1 medium cauliflower
20 g salt
White wine vinegar or cider vinegar (enough to cover the cauliflower)
1 teaspoon green peppercorns
1 teaspoon black peppercorns
1 teaspoon pink peppercorns
1–6 fresh green, red and yellow chillies according to taste (yellow chillies are optional, as they are not always available)

In a large saucepan, blanch the cauliflower in boiling, salted water for 5 minutes. Rinse under cold water, drain and pat dry with kitchen paper. Carefully cut away small florets from the main stalk and put them into a 1½-litre hermetically-sealable pickling jar. Using a stainless steel, glass or enamel saucepan, bring to the boil the white wine or cider vinegar, peppercorns and chillies and cook them for 30 seconds. Pour the vinegar mixture over the cauliflower florets in the pickling jar so that they are completely covered. Allow to cool and seal the jar tightly. Leave for 3 weeks in a cool, dark place.

VINEGARS

blackberry vinegar

Use in salad dressings or cooking.

300 g blackberries
1 teaspoon mustard powder in a small muslin bag
1 litre white wine vinegar

Wash the blackberries in cold water, trim away any stems and green parts, drain on kitchen paper, and place in a hermetically-sealable pickling jar with the mustard. Pour over the white wine vinegar and seal the jar tightly. Leave for 2 weeks in a cool, dark place. Strain and bottle the vinegar.

raspberry vinegar

250 g raspberries
1 litre red wine vinegar

Put the raspberries in a hermetically-sealable pickling jar. Pour over the red wine vinegar and seal the jar tightly. Leave for 2 months in a cool, dark place. Strain and bottle the vinegar, pressing the fruit to extract the juice.

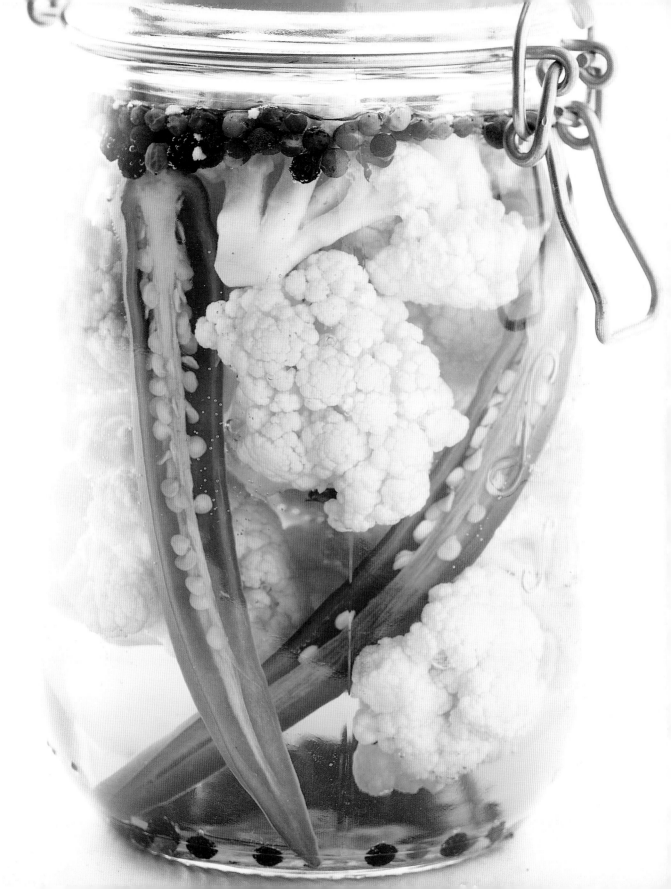

borage leaves in vinegar

The leaves can be eaten on their own as a starter or added to salads or other dishes. The borage flowers give a blue colour to the vinegar.

110 g young borage leaves
A dash of white wine vinegar
Borage flowers (10% of the volume of borage leaves)
1 litre white wine vinegar (with 2 tablespoons salt added)

Rinse the borage leaves in a bowl of cold water with a dash of vinegar added. Place the leaves in a single layer on a clean, dry cloth and leave them to wilt for 8 hours. Place them in a 1½ litre hermetically-sealable pickling jar and add the borage flowers. Pour over the salted white wine vinegar and seal the jar tightly. Leave for 1 month in a cool, dark place.

tarragon vinegar

2 handfuls fresh tarragon
10–12 very small pickling onions threaded onto toothpicks
A few borage flowers (optional)
1 litre white wine or cider vinegar

Put the tarragon into a hermetically-sealable pickling jar with the onions and the borage flowers (if using). Pour over the white wine or cider vinegar and seal the jar tightly. Leave for 2 weeks in a cool, dark place.

shallot vinegar

1 litre white wine vinegar or cider vinegar
10 shallots
1 bay leaf
1 sprig of thyme
1 teaspoon black peppercorns

Pour the white wine or cider vinegar over the other ingredients in a hermetically-sealable pickling jar. Seal the jar tightly. Leave for 2 weeks in a cool, dark place. Strain and bottle.

herb vinegar

1 litre red or white wine vinegar
1 sprig of tarragon
A few basil leaves
1 sprig of marjoram
1 sprig of thyme
1 clove (or a few juniper berries)
A few green and black peppercorns

Pour the vinegar over the other ingredients in a hermetically-sealable pickling jar. Seal the jar tightly. Leave for 1 month in a cool, dark place. Strain and bottle.

amazingly aromatic vinegar

1 litre white wine or cider vinegar
2 handfuls of tarragon leaves and stems
2 handfuls of dill
1 handful fresh basil leaves
1 handful fresh thyme
1 handful marjoram
10–12 small shallots threaded onto toothpicks
1 red chilli, whole (optional)

Pour the vinegar over the other ingredients in a hermetically-sealable pickling jar. Seal the jar tightly. Leave for 2–3 weeks in a cool, dark place. Strain and bottle, leaving the thyme in the vinegar.

table mustard

2 tablespoons chopped parsley
2 tablespoons chopped chervil
2 tablespoons chopped chives
2 tablespoons chopped celery leaves
2 tablespoons chopped tarragon
2 tablespoons chopped thyme
1 clove of garlic
1 teaspoon salt
½ teaspoon black pepper
White wine vinegar (enough to cover the herbs)
Mustard powder
Olive oil

In a food processor, blend the herbs, garlic, and salt and pepper. Transfer to a small, hermetically-sealable pickling jar and add white wine vinegar to cover. Seal the jar tightly. Leave for 1 week in a cool, dark place. Add mustard powder to make a thick paste and olive oil to create a smooth consistency. Mix well and store in a sealed container in the refrigerator.

JAM

physalis jam

1 kg physalis berries
Water
1 kg sugar

Remove the berries from their parchment skins, wash and cut them in half. Put them into a heavy-based saucepan, cover them with water and simmer for 30 minutes. Blend the berry mixture in a food processor, add the sugar and return to the heat for 30 minutes. Store in tightly-sealed jars.

medicinal drinks, tinctures and syrups

Infusions, decoctions, wines, liqueurs, tinctures and syrups provide a valuable way of administering the active ingredients of various plants, herbs and spices. Each recipe is accompanied by the recommended dosage, a brief explanation of its properties (some of the terms used are explained in the glossary; page 140) and the ailments or body systems that it is good for. See part two for more information about specific ailments and their remedies. Most of the recipes give amounts for dried herbs. If you wish to substitute fresh herbs, use two to three times the given amount. Dried herbs can be bought from health food shops and herbalists.

INFUSIONS

Infusions can be prepared one day in advance, stored in the refrigerator and gently warmed when needed. They are relatively mild medicinal drinks and need to be taken frequently. Infusions made with lime flower, lemon balm and camomile are recommended for children.

dandelion infusion

Dosage: 150 ml three times a day.
Properties: detoxifying, aids liver function.
Good for: bone and joint disorders, digestive system disorders, kidney and
        bladder disorders, eczema, high blood pressure.

1 litre boiling water
1 tablespoon dried dandelion root
1 tablespoon dried dandelion leaves

Pour the boiling water over the dandelion root and leaves, and cover. Leave to infuse for 10 minutes then strain.

fennel infusion

Dosage: 150 ml three times a day. Alternatively, take a drop of fennel
        essential oil on a lump of sugar or in a teaspoon of honey.
Properties: anti-spasmodic, carminative, appetite and digestion stimulant.
Good for: digestive system disorders, women's health disorders, anaemia,
        candida, polymyalgia rheumatica, Raynaud's disease.

150 ml boiling water
1 tablespoon fennel seeds or root

Pour the boiling water over the fennel seeds or root, and cover. Leave to infuse for 10 minutes then strain.

raspberry-leaf infusion

Dosage: 150 ml of the warm infusion three times a day.
Properties: astringent.
Good for: fibrositis, period pain, polymyalgia rheumatica, pregnancy
        (especially the last few weeks).

150 ml boiling water
1 teaspoon dried raspberry leaves

Pour the boiling water over the raspberry leaves and cover. Leave to infuse for 5 minutes then strain.

orange-zest infusion

Dosage: drink throughout the day instead of water.
Properties: stimulates the immune system.
Good for: blood and circulation disorders.

1 litre boiling water
40 g orange zest
15 g bay leaves

Pour the boiling water over the orange zest and bay leaves, and cover. Leave to infuse for 20 minutes then strain.

marjoram infusion

Dosage: drink throughout the day instead of water. For ease of use,
        mix the herbs together and store them in a jar.
Properties: aids digestion, antiseptic, anti-spasmodic.
Good for: respiratory system disorders, immune system disorders,
        insomnia, thrush.

20 g dried marjoram
20 g dried thyme
20 g dried mint
½ litre boiling water
Honey to taste

Pour the boiling water over 15 g of the herb mixture and cover. Leave to infuse for a few minutes. Strain and add honey to taste.

lemon-balm and camomile infusion *(right)*

Dosage: 150 ml of the warm infusion two or three times a day. For ease of use, mix the herbs together and store them in a jar.
Properties: antispasmodic, sedative, detoxifying.
Good for: heart and circulation disorders, digestive system disorders, respiratory system disorders, nervous system disorders, women's health disorders, kidney stones, psoriasis, urticaria (hives).

100 g dried lemon balm leaves
30 g dried camomile flowers
20 g dried mint leaves
150 ml boiling water

Pour the boiling water over a tablespoon of the herb mixture and cover. Leave to infuse for 5 minutes then strain.

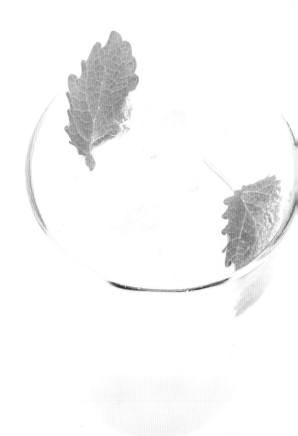

carrot-seed infusion

Dosage: 150 ml two or three times a day.
Properties: stimulates digestion, tonic, promotes bile flow, mild diuretic.
Good for: amenorrhoea.

300 ml boiling water
5 g carrot seeds

Pour the boiling water over the carrot seeds, and cover. Leave to infuse for 10 minutes then strain.

pear and apple infusion

Dosage: drink throughout the day instead of water.
Properties: diuretic, anti-inflammatory, detoxifying.
Good for: bone and joint disorders, kidney and bladder stones.

1 litre boiling water
50 g pear leaves
50 g dried apple peel

Pour the boiling water over the pear leaves and apple peel and cover. Infuse for 20 minutes and strain.

barley infusion

Dosage: drink throughout the day instead of water.
Properties: diuretic, calming, anti-inflammatory.
Good for: irritable bladder, prostatitis.

1 litre boiling water
100 g barley grain

Pour the boiling water over the barley and cover. Leave to infuse for 3 hours then strain.

elder and camomile infusion

Dosage: 150 ml of the warm infusion three or four times a day. This infusion can be given to young children.
Properties: promotes sweating, detoxifying, sedative, anti-inflammatory.
Good for: digestive system, respiratory system, nervous system, immune system, endometriosis, premenstrual syndrome, psoriasis.

250 ml boiling water
2 tablespoons dried elderflowers
1 tablespoon dried camomile flowers (or 1 camomile teabag)
Sugar to taste

Pour the boiling water over the elderflowers and camomile flowers and cover. Leave to infuse for 10 minutes. Strain and sweeten with sugar.

sparkling lemon-balm infusion

Dosage: drink when desired. This recipe can be served as an aperitif for adults by replacing the sparkling water with sparkling wine.
Properties: refreshing, calming (excellent for children).
Good for: nervous system, women's health, angina, anxiety, cough, fear and nightmares in children, laryngitis, psoriasis, rhinitis, urticaria (hives).

For the infusion:
½ litre boiling water
45 fresh lemon balm leaves

For the drink:
½ litre sparkling mineral water – or wine if using
Juice of 1 orange
Juice of 1 grapefruit
Sugar to taste
1 fresh lemon balm leaf
1 slice of lemon

Pour the boiling water over the lemon balm leaves and cover. Leave to infuse until cold and then strain. Mix the infusion with the sparkling mineral water, or wine if using, orange and grapefruit juice. Add sugar to taste and serve in a frosted glass with the lemon-balm leaf and a slice of lemon.

coriander-seed infusion

Dosage: 150 ml of the warm infusion two or three times a day.
Properties: anti-spasmodic, carminative, stimulates the digestive system.
Good for: digestive system, amenorrhoea, period pain.

150 ml boiling water
1 tablespoon coriander seeds
Sugar to taste

Pour the boiling water over the coriander seeds and cover. Leave to infuse for 10 minutes. Strain and add sugar to taste.

ginger infusion

Dosage: 150 ml of the warm infusion four times a day or when desired.
Properties: stimulates digestive system, anti-emetic.
Good for: heart and circulation, digestive system, respiratory system, nervous system, digestive problems and morning sickness during pregnancy.

150 ml boiling water
2 tablespoons grated fresh root ginger
Sugar to taste

Pour the boiling water over the ginger and cover. Allow to infuse for 5 minutes. Strain and sweeten with a little sugar.

DECOCTIONS

As with infusions, decoctions can be prepared one day in advance, they are relatively mild and should be taken frequently. Decoctions involve boiling the tough or woody parts of plants, such as stems, roots, seeds and berries. Store decoctions in the refrigerator.

carrot-leaf decoction

Usage: apply to the skin two or three times a day.
Properties: promotes healing and regeneration of damaged skin, anti-inflammatory, analgesic.
Good for: chilblains.

1 handful of fresh carrot leaves
150 ml water
Carrot juice (extracted using a juicer)

In a saucepan, boil the carrot leaves in the water for 5 minutes. Strain and mix with an equal quantity of fresh carrot juice.

cherry-stem decoction

Dosage: 150 ml three or four times a day.
Properties: diuretic, detoxifying.
Good for: bone and joint disorders, measles, pleurisy, pneumonia.

30 g cherry stems
1 litre water

In a saucepan, boil the cherry stems in the water for 10 minutes and strain.

corn-hair and fennel-seed decoction

Corn hair consists of black, hair-like threads that surround the corn beneath the outer leaves. It is available in specialist herb shops or from herbalists.

Dosage: 150 ml of the warm infusion three times a day.
Properties: detoxifying, diuretic, anti-inflammatory, stimulates the digestive system.
Good for: kidney and bladder disorders, women's health, chickenpox, prostatitis.

1 handful of dried corn hair
2 teaspoons fennel seeds
1 litre water

In a saucepan, bring the ingredients to the boil. Remove from heat, cover and leave to infuse for 20 minutes. Strain.

lychee-seed decoction

Dosage: drink the warm decoction throughout the day.
Properties: analgesic, anti-spasmodic, astringent.
Good for: abdominal cramp and colic.

30 g lychee seeds
Zest of 1 lemon
1 tablespoon fennel seeds
½ litre water

In a saucepan, boil the ingredients in the water for 20 minutes, then strain.

physalis-berry decoction

Dosage: 150 ml four times a day.
Properties: diuretic, anti-inflammatory.
Good for: kidney and bladder disorders, prostatitis.

60 g physalis berries
1 litre water

In a saucepan, boil the berries in the water for 5 minutes. Allow to infuse for a further 10 minutes and strain.

cherry-stem and apple decoction

Dosage: 150 ml three times a day.
Properties: detoxifying, anti-inflammatory, diuretic.
Good for: arthritis (rheumatoid), chickenpox, measles.

1 handful of cherry stems
1 litre water
2 or 3 apples, sliced

In a saucepan, boil the cherry stems in the water for 10 minutes. Strain and pour the decoction over the apple slices. Cover and leave to infuse for 20 minutes. Strain, pressing the apple slices to extract all the juice.

lettuce-seed decoction

Dosage: 250 ml three times a day.
Properties: calming, sedative, anti-spasmodic.
Good for: respiratory disorders, anxiety, kidney stones.

1 tablespoon lettuce seeds
250 ml water

In a saucepan, boil the lettuce seeds in the water for 10 minutes and then strain.

dill-seed decoction

Dosage: 150 ml of the warm infusion two or three times a day.
Properties: anti-spasmodic, carminative, stimulates the digestive system.
Good for: digestive system disorders, amenorrhoea, period pain.

1 tablespoon dill seeds
500 ml water
Sugar to taste

In a saucepan, boil the dill seeds in the water for 10 minutes. Strain and add sugar to taste.

fennel-seed decoction

Dosage: 150 ml of the warm infusion once a day.

Properties: anti-spasmodic, carminative, stimulates the digestive system.
Good for: digestive system disorders, women's health disorders, anaemia, polymyalgia rheumatica, Raynaud's disease.

1 dessertspoon fennel seeds
150 ml water
Sugar to taste

In a saucepan, boil the seeds in the water for 5 minutes. Strain. Add sugar.

strawberry-leaf decoction

Dosage: drink throughout the day.
Properties: astringent, anti-inflammatory, detoxifying.
Good for: bone and joint, heart and circulation, respiratory system, kidney and bladder disorders, prostatitis.

1 handful fresh strawberry leaves
1 handful fresh strawberry roots
1 litre water

In a saucepan, bring the ingredients to the boil. Remove from the heat and allow to infuse for 10 minutes. Strain.

cumin-seed decoction

Dosage: 150 ml of the warm infusion two or three times a day.
Properties: sedative, carminative, antiseptic.
Good for: digestive system, women's health.

1 teaspoon cumin seeds
150 ml water

In a saucepan, boil the cumin seeds in the water for 10 minutes. Strain.

barley water

Dosage: drink throughout the day.
Properties: diuretic, calming, anti-inflammatory.
Good for: heart and circulation, digestive system, kidney and bladder.

1 litre water
30 g barley, germinated
Honey to taste

In a saucepan, bring the water and barley gently to the boil. Simmer until the barley is cooked. Strain and add honey.

WINES AND LIQUEURS

Only small amounts of the following drinks need to be taken for medicinal purposes. Wines should be stored in tightly corked bottles and kept for a few weeks. When preparing liqueurs, use the strongest alcohol available to help to extract the plants' active ingredients. Liqueurs can last for years. Store away from bright light. Wines and liqueurs should not be given to children.

cinnamon wine *(right)*

Dosage: 50 ml when desired.
Properties: tonic, aphrodisiac, antiseptic, aids digestion.
Good for: Raynaud's disease.

50 g cinnamon bark
20 g vanilla pods
750 ml sweet red wine

Add the cinnamon and vanilla to the wine. Seal tightly and leave to macerate for 3 days. Strain through muslin and store in a tightly sealed bottle.

blackcurrant wine

Dosage: 50 ml a day.
Properties: tonic, astringent, laxative, improves vitality and digestion.
Good for: anaemia, polymyalgia rheumatica, Raynaud's disease,
　　　　　ulcerative colitis.

200 g blackcurrants
750 ml dry white wine
150 g sugar
150 ml strong alcohol (vodka, eau de vie or grappa)

Crush the blackcurrants in a large bowl and pour over the dry white wine. Seal the bowl with clingfilm and refrigerate for a week. Press and strain the mixture through muslin. Add the sugar and over a low heat, bring to simmering point. Do not allow to boil. Cool and add the strong alcohol. Store in a tightly sealed bottle and leave to age for several months.

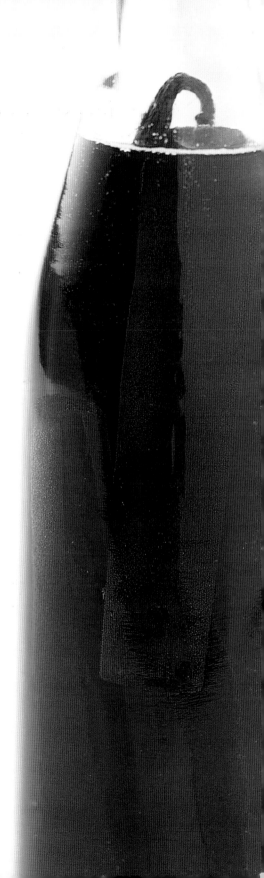

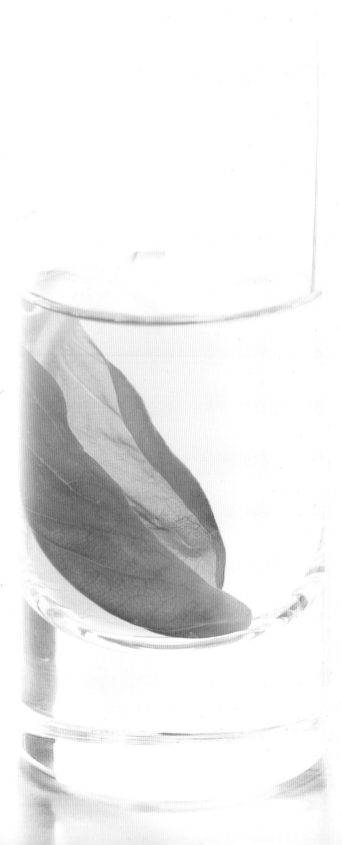

artichoke-leaf wine

Dosage: 50 ml morning and evening before meals.
Properties: detoxifying, improves liver function, stimulates the flow of bile.
Good for: ankylosing spondylitis, arteriosclerosis, cholecystitis, gallstones,
     hyperlipidaemia.

50 g dried artichoke leaves, finely chopped
750 ml red wine

Add the artichoke leaves to the wine. Seal tightly and leave to macerate for
10 days. Strain through muslin and store in a tightly sealed bottle.

cherry-leaf wine

Dosage: 50 ml a day (dilute to taste).
Properties: diuretic, detoxifying.
Good for: bone and joint disorders.

80 cherry leaves
5 tablespoons sugar
750 ml red wine
150 ml kirsch

Add the cherry leaves and the sugar to the wine. Seal tightly and leave to
macerate for 8 days. Remove the cherry leaves and add the kirsch.

blueberry wine

Dosage: 50 ml a day.
Properties: tonic, aids digestion.

200 g fresh blueberries
100 g fresh raspberries or blackcurrants
700 ml dry white wine
150 g sugar
150 ml strong alcohol (such as vodka, eau de vie or grappa)

In a large bowl, crush the fruit. Cover with the white wine, seal the bowl and
refrigerate for 1 week. Then press and strain the mixture, add the sugar to
the liquid and, in a stainless steel pan, bring to slowly to simmering point.
Cool and add the alcohol. Age in a tightly sealed bottle for several months.

juniper-berry wine

Dosage: 50 ml a day.
Properties: tonic, diuretic, analgesic, aids digestion.
Good for: kidney and bladder disorders, diabetes mellitus.

75 g fresh juniper berries, crushed
10 g lemon zest
750 ml white wine

Add the juniper berries and the lemon zest to the white wine. Seal tightly
and leave to macerate in a cool, dark place for 1 week. Strain through
muslin and store in a tightly sealed bottle.

camomile and citrus wine

Dosage: 50 ml when desired.
Properties: sedative, bitter tonic, stimulates digestion.
Good for: digestive system disorders, anxiety, endometriosis, insomnia.

60 g camomile flowers
Zest of 1 unwaxed lemon
Zest of 1 unwaxed orange
1 teaspoon tea leaves (optional)
750 ml dry white wine
60 g sugar
150 ml strong alcohol (such as vodka or gin)

Mix all the ingredients together. Seal in an airtight container and leave to macerate in a cool, dark place for 1 week. Strain through muslin and store in a tightly sealed bottle.

anisette

Dosage: 1 tablespoon (neat or diluted in 75 ml water) when desired.
Properties: anti-spasmodic, carminative.
Good for: digestive system disorders, women's health disorders, headaches and migraine.

25 g green anise seeds or star anise
15 g coriander seeds
½ g mace
1 g cinnamon bark
700 ml vodka
250 g sugar
100 ml water

Add the anise, coriander seeds, mace and cinnamon bark to the vodka. Seal tightly and leave to macerate in a cool, dark place for 1 month. In a saucepan over a low heat, completely dissolve the sugar in the water, then boil for 30 seconds. Allow to cool. Strain the vodka through muslin, pressing the seeds to extract as much liquid as possible. Mix with the cooled syrup, store in a tightly sealed bottle and keep in a cool, dark place for 2 weeks before using.

camomile aperitif

Dosage: 50 ml in the evening.
Properties: sedative, bitter tonic, enhances digestion and sleep.
Good for: endometriosis.

60 g camomile flowers
750 ml white wine

Add the camomile flowers to the wine. Seal tightly and leave to macerate in a cool, dark place for 1 month. Strain through muslin and store in a tightly sealed bottle.

lemon liqueur

Dosage: 25 ml when desired.
Properties: carminative, aids digestion, astringent, aperi
Good for: cholecystitis, gallstones.

Zest of 3 lemons, cut into thin strips
50 g almonds
1 small vanilla pod or cinnamon stick
700 ml strong vodka
250 g sugar
100 ml water
1 almond or clove

Add the lemon zest, almonds and vanilla to the vodka. Seal tightly and leave to macerate in a cool, dark place for 1 month. In a heavy-based pan, dissolve the sugar in the water completely and then boil for 30 seconds. Strain the infused alcohol and combine with the cooled syrup. Add an almond or clove and some of the original lemon zest to the mixture. Seal tightly and leave to mature for a few months.

basil liqueur *(far left)*

Dosage: 25 ml when desired.
Properties: antiseptic, anti-spasmodic, stimulates appetite.
Good for: digestive system disorders, headaches and migraine.

80 fresh basil leaves
700 ml strong vodka
250 g sugar
100 ml water

Add the basil leaves to the vodka. Seal tightly and leave to macerate in a cool dark place for 1 month. In a heavy-based pan, dissolve the sugar over a low heat in just enough water to make it wet. When all the crystals have dissolved, boil for 30 seconds. Mix the cooled syrup with the vodka, seal tightly and leave for a further 3 weeks. To keep the green colour of the liqueur remove some of the basil leaves (they can be used to make basil ice cream in an ice-cream maker).

quince liqueur

Dosage: 50 ml when desired.
Properties: astringent.
Good for: digestive system disorders.

1 kg quince, mashed
200 g sugar
2 cloves
Pinch ground cinnamon
Vodka or brandy (see method for quantity)

Refrigerate the mashed quince for 48 hours, then press through muslin to extract the juice. Add the sugar, cloves and cinnamon and an equal volume of vodka or brandy. Seal tightly and leave to macerate for 2 months. Strain through muslin and store in a tightly sealed bottle. Leave to age for a further 2 or 3 months.

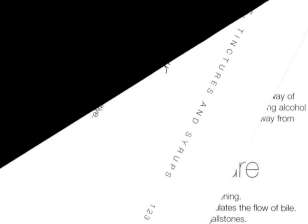

...ay of
...ng alcohol
...way from

...re

...ning.
...ulates the flow of bile.
...allstones.

...
750 m...

Add the artichoke ...   ...al tightly and leave to macerate
in a cool, dark place fo...   ...hrough muslin and store in a
tightly sealed bottle away fro...   ...t.

aniseed tincture

Dosage: 20 drops in 150 ml of water one to three times a day.
        Or take 10 drops of tincture on a lump of sugar.
Properties: anti-spasmodic, carminative, stimulates the digestive system.
Good for: digestive system disorders, women's health disorders, headaches
        and migraine.

170 g aniseed (the seeds of the anise plant)
700 ml strong alcohol (vodka, eau de vie or gin)

Add the aniseed to the alcohol. Seal tightly and leave to macerate in a cool,
dark place for 1 month. Strain through muslin and store in a tightly sealed
bottle away from bright light.

coriander-seed tincture

Dosage: 15 drops in 75 ml of water after a meal.
Properties: anti-spasmodic, carminative, aids digestion, aids lactation.
Good for: gastritis, amenorrhoea.

5 g coriander seeds
500 ml strong alcohol (vodka, gin or brandy)

Add the coriander seeds to the alcohol. Seal tightly and leave to macerate
in a cool, dark place for 1 week. Strain through muslin and store in a tightly
sealed bottle away from bright light.

SYRUPS

The active ingredients of plants can be administered in the form of a syrup.
Syrups should always be stored in a refrigerator and used within a few days
(except crème de cassis, which will keep for several months).
        The following test can help to determine the point during preparation at
which a syrup should be removed from the heat: take a teaspoon of the
syrup and drop it into a glass of cold water; if it breaks into droplets, it
needs further boiling; if it forms a single droplet, it is ready.

leek syrup

Dosage: 1 tablespoon three times a day.
Properties: soothing, expectorant, anti-inflammatory.
Good for: respiratory system disorders, fibrositis, polymyalgia rheumatica,
        sore throat, tonsillitis.

1 medium leek, chopped
1 litre water
150 g sugar

In a saucepan, simmer the leek in the water. When the water has reduced
by approximately one-third, press the leek to squeeze out the juice.
Remove the leek, add the sugar and boil for a few more minutes. Allow
to cool and pour into a sterilized bottle. Seal tightly and refrigerate.

peach syrup

Dosage: 3–4 tablespoons a day (2 tablespoons for children).
Properties: calming, laxative.
Good for: constipation in children.

150 ml boiling water
20 g fresh peach flowers
250 g honey

In a saucepan, pour the boiling water over the flowers, cover and leave to
infuse for about 6 hours. Strain through muslin, add the honey, then bring
to the boil, reduce the heat and simmer for a few minutes. Allow to cool
and pour into a sterilized bottle. Seal tightly and refrigerate.

black radish syrup

Dosage: 1 tablespoon three times a day.
Properties: soothing, anti-inflammatory, expectorant.
Good for: sore throat, tonsillitis, whooping cough.

1 black radish, peeled and sliced
Caster sugar

Place the radish slices in a dish, covering each layer with plenty of sugar.
Cover with cling film and leave overnight. Press the radish slices to extract
the syrup and strain into a sterilized bottle. Seal tightly and refrigerate.

mint syrup

Dosage: 1 teaspoon in a glass of water. Mint syrup can be added to water
or served with sorbet.
Properties: stimulates the digestive system, anti-spasmodic.
Good for: colitis, cough, endometriosis, food poisoning, rhinitis.

1 litre boiling water
100 g fresh mint leaves
1 kg sugar

Pour the water over the mint leaves. Seal tightly and leave to infuse for 24
hours. Strain. In a pan, bring the infusion and sugar to the boil and simmer
for 3 minutes. Cool. Pour into a sterilized bottle. Seal tightly and refrigerate.

blackberry syrup *(right)*

Dosage: 1 tablespoon in 150 ml of water two or three times a day.
Properties: astringent.
Good for: diarrhoea, dysentery.

1 kg blackberries
1 kg sugar
150 ml water

In a pan, bring the ingredients to the boil. Reduce the heat and simmer for
10 minutes. Cool. Pour into a sterilized bottle. Seal tightly and refrigerate.

crème de cassis

Dosage: take as desired. This vitamin C-rich syrup can be diluted with
water for children or added to dry white wine for adults.
Properties: tonic.
Good for: general well-being.

6 kg blackcurrants
6 kg sugar

Fill up 1 kg jars with equal amounts of blackcurrants and sugar in
thin, alternating layers. Seal the jars and leave in a cool, dark place for
6 months. Strain and pour into sterilized bottles. Seal tightly and refrigerate.

asparagus syrup

Dosage: 2 tablespoons morning and evening.
Properties: diuretic and sedative.
Good for: nervous system disorders, endometriosis, palpitations,
premenstrual syndrome, psoriasis.

200 ml asparagus tips juice (extracted using a juicer)
400 g sugar

In a saucepan, boil the asparagus juice and sugar until a thick syrup forms.
Allow to cool and pour into a sterilized bottle. Seal tightly and refrigerate.

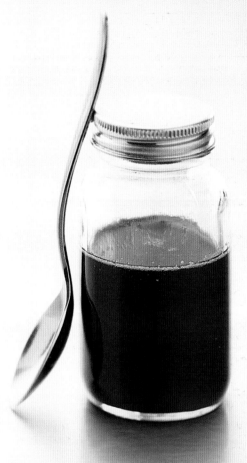

elderberry syrup

Dosage: 1 tablespoon every morning.
Properties: gentle laxative.
Good for: colic, constipation, irritable bowel syndrome (recommended for
elderly people).

1½ kg fresh elderberries, slightly unripe (red rather than black), with the
stems cut off
150 ml water
350 g sugar
3 g cloves

In a saucepan, crush the berries and simmer them in the water for
30 minutes. Put the berry mixture in a piece of muslin and allow the juice
to drip into a bowl overnight. In a non-reactive saucepan, bring the juice,
sugar and cloves to the boil. Reduce the heat and simmer for 5 minutes.
Allow to cool and pour into a sterilized bottle. Seal tightly and refrigerate.

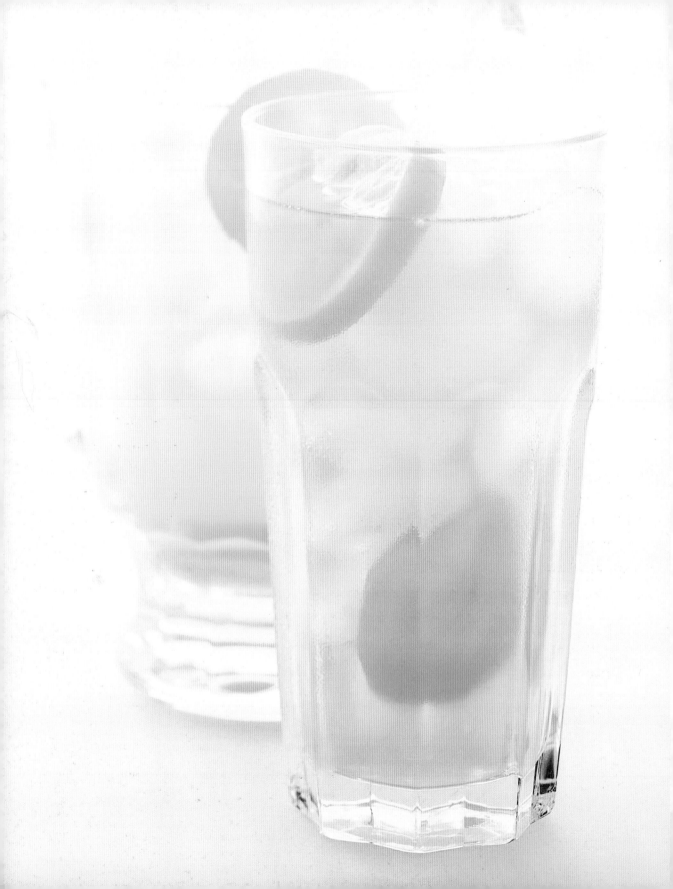

diet in practice

Sometimes the best way to fortify the body against illness is to simplify the diet to a few basic ingredients that are easy to digest and assimilate. This enables the body to rid itself of toxins and emerge stronger and more resilient. The detoxification programme on the following pages – a four-week prescription of healing foods, drinks and exercise – is the ideal way to accomplish this. It can be followed successfully by most adults regardless of their level of health and fitness. This part of the book also presents the vitamins, minerals and other nutrients, such as antioxidants and essential fatty acids, that are needed for health, together with a selection of the foods in which they are found. There is also a short review of two basic elements of our everyday diet that have important health-giving properties but are often overlooked: culinary oils and bottled mineral waters.

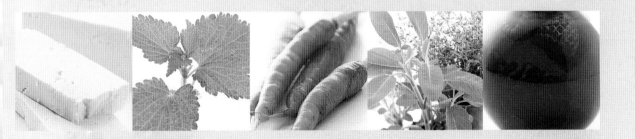

the detox programme

During digestion, a certain amount of acids are produced – these are partly a result of normal digestive processes and partly a result of the incomplete degradation of animal proteins. The body gets rid of a small amount of these acids rapidly via the lungs but denser acids, such as uric, phosphoric and sulphuric acid, which are generated by the breakdown of animal protein, are eliminated slowly by the kidneys. If acid is not eliminated quickly enough, it creates toxicity.

A series of complex operations involving a variety of secretions – each acting under different pH – takes place in the digestive tract. The result of these operations is the breakdown of food into nutrients that can be used by the body. However, if the pH in one section of the gut is wrong, the digestive process is impaired and fats, sugars and proteins are only partially broken down. Food starts to putrefy in the gut and a pathogenic flora develops to the detriment of the beneficial flora. This also creates toxicity in the body.

According to the late Dr Kousmine, a nutrition and cancer specialist, acids that are not eliminated from the body during the day are stored in extra-cellular fluid (known as serous fluid) in the peritoneum. At night when the body is resting the acids are filtered and disposed of. Over a period of time, however, acids build up in the body's tissues causing an accumulation of toxins and a condition known as chronic acidosis. This can give rise to a variety of symptoms including fatigue, disturbed sleep, regurgitation, heartburn, lack of appetite or bulimia, diarrhoea or constipation, migraine, bad breath, cold perspiration, lowered resistance to infections, muscular pain, rheumatism, bronchitis and excessive mucus production resulting in chronic catarrh.

In the past 50 years, there has been an increase in heart disease, cancer and auto-immune or degenerative disorders such as rheumatoid arthritis. Rather than having mechanical, bacterial or viral causes, these illnesses are directly or indirectly linked to food processing and preserving methods and the excessive consumption of refined sugar, cereals, oils, meat, dairy and animal fat. The use of hormones, chemical fertilizers, antibiotics, insecticides and anti-fungal agents has also contributed to the build-up of toxins in the food chain.

A detoxification diet can facilitate the rapid and efficient elimination of toxins and improve both short- and long-term health. The plan described here combines diet and exercise with herbal medicine and nutritional supplements. Although it is suitable for the majority of adults, it should not be followed by children, elderly people or pregnant or breastfeeding women. If you are on long-term medication, such as hormone replacement therapy (HRT), or drugs for hypertension or thyroid problems, you should continue to take them throughout the programme (consult your doctor if you are in any doubt about whether it is safe for you to follow a detox plan). It is useful to be aware of some possible side-effects of detoxification. These vary depending on the stage of the programme but they tend to include mild headache, mood changes and energy fluctuations. If side effects do not abate after the first week, or you experience persistent or troublesome symptoms, consult your doctor.

Although the detox plan requires a few changes to your normal routine and some careful planning, it should be fairly easy to implement. Most people start to feel the benefits of detox about 10 days into the programme.

week one

WHAT TO DO

During the first week you should eliminate all dairy and wheat-based products from your diet, reduce your salt intake, avoid meat and animal fat, tea, coffee, white sugar, sweets, alcohol and tobacco. Remember that foods such as pasta, biscuits and bread all contain wheat; use rice, buckwheat or quinoa as a substitute. Soya milk is readily available and can be used as a replacement for cow's milk. In addition, you should:

● Drink 1–2 litres of mineral water every day; choose water that has a low mineral content (page 138).

● If you experience an excessive amount of abdominal gas and bloating, take two capsules of activated charcoal three times a day after meals.

● Eat a handful of fresh or dried blueberries every day.

● Drink herbal teas made from fennel, ginger or camomile before and after your meals.

● Use plenty of herbs such as thyme, basil, rosemary, garlic and shallots in your cooking.

HOW TO SUCCEED

● Revise your usual shopping list to include plenty of fresh fruit and vegetables, fish, rice, lentils, beans, millet, buckwheat flour, fresh herbs and herbal teas such as ginger, peppermint, camomile and fennel.

● Follow the recipes in this book and use a cookery book with an emphasis on healthy food (Provençal and Mediterranean cooking are recommended).

● Start the day with a protein-based breakfast (mushrooms are a good source of protein) and eat well at lunchtime. This will provide you with enough energy to get through the day. In contrast, your dinner should be very light.

● Resist the temptation to have the occasional sugary snack, cup of tea or coffee or alcoholic drink.

POSSIBLE SIDE-EFFECTS

You may experience mild headaches, bursts of energy alternating with fatigue, muscle aches and pains, sudden hunger, irritability, cravings for sweet foods, intestinal gas, abdominal distension, and regurgitation. These are most common during the first 48 hours. Side-effects vary from one person to another and you certainly won't experience all of these.

THE BENEFITS

Towards the end of week one, you may notice that your energy levels, appetite and quality of sleep are improving.

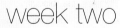

week two

WHAT TO DO

Follow exactly the same guidelines as for week one but increase the percentage of raw fruit and vegetables so that they make up 70 per cent of your daily food intake. In addition, avoid eating after seven o'clock in the evening.

● To accelerate the detoxification process, drink 150 ml dandelion infusion (page 117), three times a day. Or drink 50 ml artichoke leaf wine (page 122) at lunchtime and early evening.

● Take propolis tablets to help reduce bacterial activity in the gut. Follow the dosage instructions on the package.

HOW TO SUCCEED

● Drink as much herbal tea as you like after seven o'clock in the evening.

● Try to go to bed earlier than usual – rest is an important aid to detoxification.

● Keep following the tips for success for week one.

POSSIBLE SIDE-EFFECTS

Cravings for sweets and carbohydrates and feelings of hunger are common during week two. You may feel tired or cold immediately after you have had a meal and you may start to lose weight.

THE BENEFITS

Towards the end of week two you will start to feel more energetic both physically and mentally. Your digestion, breathing and sleep patterns will be better and you may start to notice an improvement in chronic conditions, such as poor skin, eczema, rheumatism or arthritis.

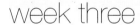

week three

WHAT TO DO

You should continue the programme of diet and rest that you followed in week two but, to accelerate detoxification, you should build in a programme of daily exercise. Do some low intensity exercise for 45 minutes twice daily. The best types of exercise are brisk walking, cycling or swimming.

You should also step up your intake of vitamins, minerals and trace elements by drinking a glass of fruit or vegetable juice twice every day. Recommended fruit juices are carrot, blackberry, blueberry, cherry or apricot. Good vegetable juice combinations include broccoli, green bean and lemon juice or carrot, cabbage and green or red pepper.

Before breakfast in the morning, drink the juice of half a lemon mixed with an equal amount of cold-pressed olive oil. This combination facilitates the emulsion and flow of bile into the digestive system. Other important dietary measures for week three are:

● Eat more of the following foods: rice, root vegetables such as carrot, celeriac, Jerusalem artichoke and turnip, germinated pulses, green vegetables, raw apple, fig and brazil nut.

● Eat fish at least twice a week.

● Drink 1–2 litres of mineral water every day; preferably with a medium to high mineral content (page 138).

HOW TO SUCCEED

● Drink some water or herbal tea before you exercise, but avoid exercising on a full stomach.

● Eat a light snack after exercise, but nothing too heavy.

● Keep following the tips for success for weeks one and two.

POSSIBLE SIDE-EFFECTS

Weight loss will continue as you burn calories during exercise. Exercise may also give rise to symptoms such as muscular aches (a recommended remedy for this is homeopathic arnica tablets of 30 or 200 potency; take when needed). However, if you experience a strong tightening or gripping pain in the centre of your chest after a few minutes of exercise, you must rest immediately and consult your doctor. Any sharp pains in weight-bearing joints or your lower back, should also be reported to your doctor.

THE BENEFITS

You should continue to experience the benefits described in week 2. You will continue to feel more energetic, and your digestion, breathing and sleep patterns will improve further.

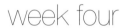

week four

WHAT TO DO

Continue to follow a wheat- and dairy-free diet but reduce your raw fruit and vegetable consumption to 50 per cent of your total food intake. Start to eat lightly after 7 pm. Continue your twice-daily exercise programme and keep taking the olive oil and lemon juice mixture before breakfast as in week 3. Drink fruit or vegetable juice twice a day and at least 1½ litres of a mineral water that has a medium-to-high mineral content.

HOW TO SUCCEED

● Take a fish oil supplement every day for the next few weeks.

● Keep following the tips for success for weeks one to three.

POSSIBLE SIDE-EFFECTS

At this stage of your programme, you should not experience any noticeable side-effects.

THE BENEFITS

You should be feeling really fit and healthy by week four. Your energy levels should be consistently high, you should be sleeping well and any minor digestive problems should have completely disappeared. Chronic conditions such as eczema or rheumatism should be more manageable and may even have disappeared. Your immune system will be stronger and you will be more resistant to colds and influenza.

your diet after detox

Once you have completed your four-week detoxification programme you can either follow the week-four guidelines for a further two weeks or you can return to a normal diet.

If you return to a normal diet, gradually reintroduce wheat products in the first week. If you experience any symptoms in response to them, eliminate wheat from your diet permanently. Dairy products should be reintroduced during the second week and any symptoms monitored. Again, if you have an adverse response, eliminate dairy products from your diet permanently.

Continue to practise as many aspects of the detox diet as you can and make sure that you apply the following principles to your long-term diet and lifestyle:

● Keep drinking plenty of water. Drink mineral water with a low mineral content (page 138), unless advised and supervised by a doctor or nutritionist.

● Eat meat and drink wine, coffee and tea in moderation.

● Keep up your exercise programme.

● Follow the detox programme annually and repeat the first two weeks of the plan twice a year: once in the autumn and once in the spring.

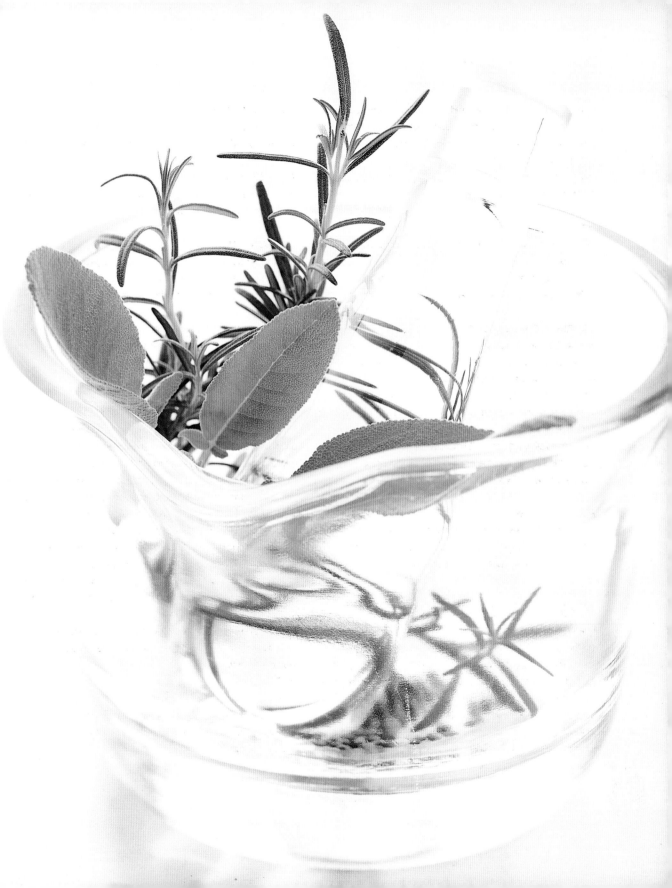

directory of vitamins, minerals and other nutrients

THIS CHART LISTS VITAMINS, MINERALS AND OTHER NUTRIENTS THAT FORM AN IMPORTANT PART OF OUR DIET. THE BENEFITS OF EACH ARE GIVEN, AS WELL AS EXAMPLES OF FOODS THAT ARE PARTICULARLY GOOD SOURCES OF A NUTRIENT.

VITAMIN	BENEFITS	SOURCES
VITAMIN A (Retinol)	Vitamin A is important for maintaining healthy skin. It also helps prevent frequent infections of the upper respiratory tract, such as colds and sore throats, and improves night vision. Retinol is found in animal products but vitamin A can also be produced from carotenes found in plant foods.	● carrot (pages 14–15) ● watercress (page 17) ● cabbage (pages 18–19) ● mango (page 30) ● melon (page 32)
VITAMIN B1 (Thiamine)	Vitamin B1 increases concentration. It is easily destroyed by cooking or exposure to ultra-violet light. A low intake of vitamin B1 can cause depression and irritability.	● watercress (page 17) ● cabbage (pages 18–19) ● courgette (page 20)
VITAMIN B2 (Riboflavin)	Vitamin B2 is essential for the metabolism of fats, sugars and proteins in the body.	● watercress (page 17) ● cabbage (pages 18–19) ● asparagus (page 23) ● milk (page 55)
VITAMIN B3 (Niacin)	Vitamin B3 reinforces the skin's natural protection against exposure to the sun. Deficiency can cause fatigue, depression, poor concentration and dermatitis.	● cabbage (pages 18–19) ● courgette (page 20)
VITAMIN B5 (Pantothenic acid)	Vitamin B5 is important for the health of the immune system and helps the body extract energy from food.	● watercress (page 17) ● cabbage (pages 18–19) ● celery (page 20) ● avocado (page 23) ● strawberry (page 33)

VITAMIN	BENEFITS	SOURCES
VITAMIN B6 (Pyridoxine)	Vitamin B6 is necessary for healthy blood and for the metabolization of protein.	● onion (page 12) ● watercress (page 17) ● cabbage (pages 18–19) ● banana (page 30)
VITAMIN B12	Vitamin B12 is needed for the health of the nerves and to make red blood cells. Low intake can cause fatigue and dry skin.	● milk and cheese (page 55) ● egg (page 55)
BIOTIN	Biotin plays an important part in the metabolism of carbohydrate and fat.	● cabbage (pages 18–19) ● cherry (page 33) ● grapefruit (page 37) ● milk (page 55) ● egg (page 55)
FOLATE (folic acid; part of the vitamin B complex)	Folate is crucial for making genetic material and red blood cells. Women should take 400 mcg of folate daily during pregnancy.	● broccoli (page 16) ● cauliflower (page 16)
VITAMIN C	Vitamin C promotes tissue repair and wound-healing and is important for the general health of the immune system. It is an antioxidant and plays a major role in the absorption of iron and the formation of antibodies and collagen.	● broccoli (page 16) ● cabbage (pages 18–19) ● pepper (page 20) ● lemon (pages 38–39)
VITAMIN D (Calciferol)	Vitamin D is essential for healthy bones and skin. Sunlight is our main source of this vitamin, although low levels are present in some foods. When the skin is in contact with sunlight it manufactures its own vitamin D.	● lettuce (page 17) ● date (page 30) ● cottage cheese (page 55) ● egg (page 55)
VITAMIN E (Tocopherol)	A powerful antioxidant, vitamin E prevents the degeneration of nerves and muscles. It helps keep the skin healthy and helps to prevent cardiovascular disease.	● wheat (page 27) ● peanut (page 41)

MINERAL	BENEFITS	SOURCES
CALCIUM	A major constituent of bone and teeth, calcium is also vital to nerve transmission, blood clotting and muscle function. It regulates the heartbeat and helps maintain a proper acid-alkaline balance. A good calcium intake is also important for healthy skin.	● seaweed (page 23) ● prune (page 32) ● almond (page 41) ● milk, cheese, butter, yoghurt (page 55)
COPPER	Copper is a trace element that is vital in forming connective tissue and for the growth of healthy bones. It helps the body absorb iron from food and is present in many enzymes, which protect against free radical damage.	● fig (page 30)
FLUORIDE	This mineral protects against tooth decay.	● asparagus (page 23)
IODINE	Iodine is required by the thyroid gland in order to produce the thyroid hormone, which regulates physical and mental development, including growth, reproduction and many other essential functions.	● barley (page 27) ● banana (page 30) ● grape and raisin (page 32) ● shellfish (page 55) ● egg (page 55)
IRON	Essential for the production of haemoglobin, the pigment in red blood cells that transports oxygen to every cell, iron also boosts energy levels, prevents anaemia and increases the body's resistance to disease.	● bean (page 24) ● lentil (page 24) ● prune (page 32) ● walnut (page 41) ● parsley (page 43)
MAGNESIUM	Magnesium is an important constituent of bones and teeth and is important for muscle contraction. It also calms the nervous system and regulates the heartbeat. It is required for normal calcium function.	● hazelnut (page 41) ● almond (page 41) ● pine nut (page 41) ● walnut (page 41)

MINERAL	BENEFITS	SOURCES
PHOSPHORUS	Phosphorus regulates protein activity and is essential for the release of energy in the body's cells. It also helps to form and maintain healthy bones and teeth and is necessary for the absorption of many nutrients.	● present in most foods
POTASSIUM	Potassium has a variety of functions: it regulates body fluids; it is essential for correct functioning of the cells and the transmission of nerve impulses; it keeps the heartbeat regular and maintains normal blood pressure.	● cauliflower (page 16) ● cabbage (pages 18–19) ● celery (page 20) ● mushroom (page 24)
SELENIUM	An antioxidant that protects from heart disease, some cancers and premature aging, selenium is required for normal growth and fertility, thyroid action, proper liver function and healthy skin and hair.	● mushroom (page 24) ● buckwheat (page 25) ● walnut (page 41) ● shellfish (page 55) ● egg (page 55)
SILICA	Vital to the development of bones, silica also promotes healthy skin and connective tissues.	● leek (page 13) ● green bean (page 16) ● nettle (page 16) ● chickpea (page 25) ● strawberry (page 33)
SODIUM	Sodium regulates the balance of body fluids and controls levels of electrolytes in blood plasma. It is essential for nerve and muscle function. Most people in the Western world consume far more sodium than they need.	● seaweed (page 23) ● oat (page 27) ● grape and raisin (page 32)
SULPHUR	In its pure form sulphur works as an antifungal and antibacterial agent – it is used in creams for treating skin disorders such as acne. Sulphur also helps form proteins. It is present in every cell.	● radish (page 13) ● cucumber (page 20) ● fennel (page 23) ● mango (page 30) ● horseradish (page 50)
ZINC	Zinc benefits the reproductive system, fertility and the skin. It also helps wounds to heal and regulates the sense of taste. Zinc is required for a healthy immune system and good night vision and is vital for normal growth.	● red meat (page 55) ● shellfish (page 55) ● egg (page 55)

OTHER NUTRIENTS	BENEFITS	SOURCES
ALLIUM COMPOUNDS	Allium compounds aid the proper function of the cardiovascular and immune systems.	● onion and shallot (page 12) ● leek (page 13) ● chive (page 44) ● garlic (pages 48–49)
ALPHA-LINOLEIC ACID	This is an essential fatty acid that is also known as omega-3 fatty acid. It has an anti-inflammatory effect that makes it good for rheumatoid arthritis, it helps to lower blood pressure and cholesterol, and reduce the likelihood of blood clots and heart attacks. It maintains cell membranes and transports fats around the body.	● oily fish (pages 56–57)
ANTHOCYANOSIDES	These antioxidants inhibit a variety of dangerous bacteria including E. coli.	● blueberry (pages 34–35)
BIOFLAVONOIDS	Bioflavonoids are antioxidants that facilitate the absorption of vitamin C. They strengthen the capillaries, which improves poor circulation and helps to prevent cardiovascular disease.	● blueberry (pages 34–35) ● mandarin and tangerine (page 37) ● grapefruit (page 37)
CAPSAICIN	An antioxidant, capsaicin can act as a pain reliever and anti-inflammatory agent. It also helps to reduce blood cholesterol and the risk of blood clots, aids digestion and may kill harmful bacteria. Capsaicin may also prevent DNA damage.	● chilli (page 46)
CAROTENOIDS (CAROTENE)	Carotenoids give the orange or yellow colour to vegetables such as carrots. They have antioxidant properties that help to prevent cellular damage caused by free-radical attack. They also reduce the risk of cancer and cardiovascular disease.	● carrot (pages 14–15) ● spinach (page 17) ● pumpkin (page 24) ● mango (page 30)

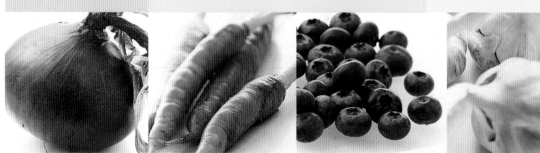

OTHER NUTRIENTS	BENEFITS	SOURCES
CHLOROPHYLL	Chlorophyll is the substance that gives plants their characteristic green colour. It is thought to help keep blood healthy, promote wound healing and kill bacteria. It may provide some protection against cancer and certain forms of radiation.	● green bean (page 16) ● dandelion (page 16) ● lamb's lettuce (page 17) ● rocket (page 17) ● sorrel (page 45)
ELLAGIC ACID	A flavonoid found in fruits, ellagic acid appears directly to protect genes from attack by carcinogens.	● cherry (page 33)
GAMMA-LINOLEIC ACID	By helping to keep the blood thin, gamma-linoleic acid contributes to the prevention of blood clots and blockages. It also reduces inflammation and relieves pain and improves nervous- and immune-system function.	● borage oil (page 45)
LINOLEIC ACID	This essential fatty acid is also known as omega-6 fatty acid. It can help to lower blood cholesterol.	● olive (pages 28–29) ● sunflower seed (page 51) ● walnut (page 41)
MALIC ACID	Malic acid makes it possible for the body to convert sugars and fats into energy.	● apple (page 37)
OLEIC ACID	High levels of oleic acid can lower cholesterol levels.	● olive (pages 28–29)
PECTIN	Pectin lowers blood pressure and blood cholesterol, softens stools to help prevent bulges in the colon and haemorrhoids, and reduces the risk of colon cancer.	● orange (page 33) ● apple (page 37) ● pear (page 37) ● persimmon (page 37) ● quince (page 37)
PHYTOESTROGEN	May help to alleviate menopausal symptoms and lower the risk of breast cancer. Mimics the activity of oestrogen in the body.	● soya beans (page 25)

mineral water and culinary oils

water

Water is essential to life in any form. It makes up approximately two-thirds of the human body and is constantly being lost in the form of sweat, water vapour, urine and faeces. We need to replace this by drinking 1–2 litres water every day.

Water varies greatly in content. The quality of the tap water in large urban areas is often poor. It may have been recycled three or four times and contain traces of hormones, nitrates and metals such as lead (lead pipes are still common in many old houses). Bottled mineral water is significantly richer than tap water in a range of minerals including calcium, magnesium, potassium, bicarbonate, chloride, sulphate, silica, fluoride, zinc, manganese, selenium and borate (check for these minerals on the label). Once opened, bottled water should be stored in the refrigerator and drunk quickly; it can rapidly become a breeding ground for bacteria. Some mineral waters are inappropriate for long-term daily use due to their high mineral content.

● Bottled waters with a low mineral content are excellent for every-day use and can be given to infants. They include Volvic and Evian.

● Bottled waters with a medium mineral content are beneficial when used every day for a limited amount of time. They include Vittel and Contrex. Mineral waters that are rich in calcium (San Pellegrino and Contrex) are recommended for the kidneys. Those rich in magnesium (Badoit and Hepar) are better for the liver.

● Bottled waters with a high mineral content, such as Vichy, have a stronger therapeutic action and should be drunk occasionally or as part of the detox programme (pages 128–31): they are diuretic, facilitate the elimination of toxins, strengthen teeth and bones and improve kidney and liver function. They are often recommended for rheumatism and arthritis, circulatory disorders, hypertension, low immunity, kidney problems, and digestive and metabolic problems.

culinary oils

When selecting culinary oils try to choose cold-pressed ones which are made by simple mechanical cleaning and crushing processes and retain their nutritional and therapeutic properties. Industrially extracted oils have a longer shelf-life, but have lost most of their taste and therapeutic qualities. Industrial extraction is lengthy, complicated and involves chemical processing and heating the oil to high temperatures. Recent research suggests that the industrial manipulation of fatty acids may make these oils detrimental to our health. The most common culinary oils are:

● Olive oil: in my opinion, this is the most nutritional and therapeutic type of oil (page 28).

● Sunflower oil: this is rich in vitamin E, oleic and linoleic acid. It can be used for cooking and in salads. Sunflower and walnut oil are excellent in combination – the sunflower oil moderates the strong taste of walnut and increases the shelf-life; the walnut oil supplies alpha-linoleic acid.

● Corn oil: this is rich in polyunsaturated fat (see Corn, page 25).

● Walnut oil: a mineral-rich, strong-tasting oil favoured in south-west France. It is best diluted with sunflower or corn oil. A tablespoon can be added to vegetable juices to enhance their taste and therapeutic value.

● Hazelnut oil: this has a delicate taste, is very nutritious and is best used in salads. Both hazelnut and walnut oils are traditionally given to children to support their growth and to treat mild digestive problems and worms, including tapeworm.

● Peanut oil: this can stand very high temperatures which makes it good for frying. It is of little therapeutic or nutritional value. Organic peanut oil is difficult to find.

● Sesame oil: widely used in Asian countries, this oil is comparable to olive oil in its therapeutic and nutritional value.

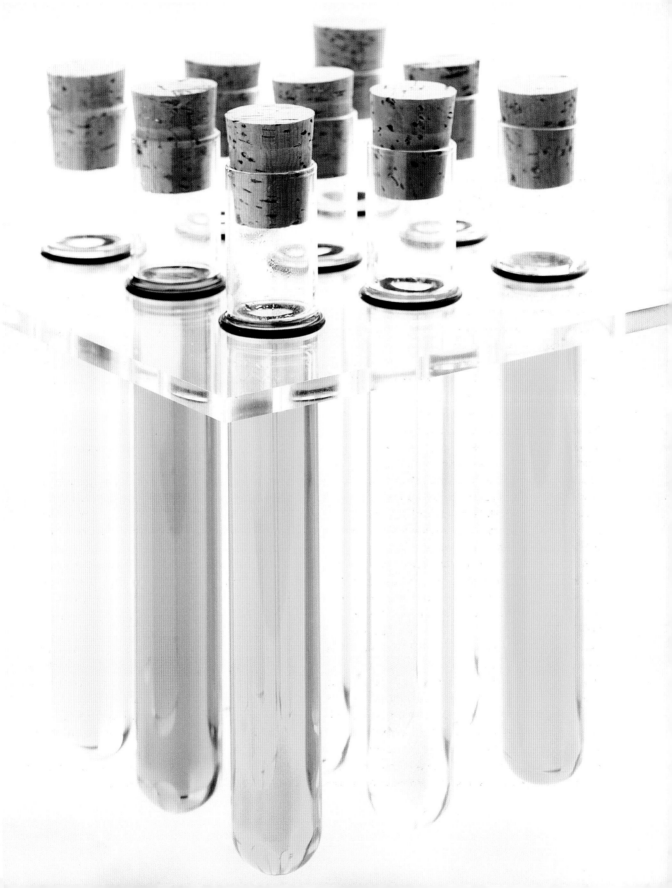

glossary

ANALGESIC ability to relieve pain.

ANTACID substance that prevents or corrects acidity.

ANTIOXIDANT substance that inhibits and controls the harmful action of free radicals. Beta-carotene, vitamins C and E, zinc and selenium are important antioxidants.

ANTI-SPASMODIC ability to prevent or reduce spasms or convulsions.

ASTRINGENT ability to promote the contraction of tissues and reduce secretions. Astringent foods cause the gut to contract, reducing permeability.

BACTERICIDAL ability to destroy bacteria.

BETAINE HYDROCHLORIDE substance that helps to facilitate digestion by contributing to gastric acidity.

BIOFLAVONOIDS group of pigments that have antioxidant properties. Found in red, green, yellow or purple fruit and vegetables.

BITTER PRINCIPLE generic name for various chemicals that are found in small quantities in some plants, such as artichokes and dandelions. Thought to be beneficial to the liver.

BROMELAIN substance found in pineapple that breaks down proteins and reduces inflammation.

CAPSAICIN substance found in hot peppers that is good for the heart and circulation.

CARMINATIVE ability to relieve flatulence.

CARDIOTONIC beneficial to the cardiovascular system.

CAROTENES group of red, orange and yellow pigments found in fruit and vegetables. Some carotenes, including alpha and beta carotenes, are transformed into vitamin A in the liver. Carotenes are antioxidants.

CHLOROPHYLL green pigment, found in plants, that has health-giving properties.

CITRIC ACID acid, found in citrus fruits, which functions as an antioxidant.

COLLAGEN main protein found in bone and connective tissue.

CRUCIFEROUS VEGETABLES family of vegetables, including broccoli and cabbage, that may help to protect against some forms of cancer.

DECOCTION concentrated solution produced by boiling a substance in water. Often used medicinally.

DEPURATIVE ability to cleanse the body or purify the blood.

DIURETIC substance that increases the flow of urine.

ELLAGIC ACID substance found in strawberries, grapes and apples that helps to prevent haemorrhage and has anti-cancer properties.

ESSENTIAL OILS complex aromatic compounds, found in a variety of plants, that have a range of therapeutic uses.

EXPECTORANT substance that promotes the movement of phlegm from the lungs through the air passages into the mouth.

FREE RADICALS harmful agents produced in the body as a result of oxidation. Have been linked to a range of age-related diseases and cancer.

GLUTEN glue-like substance found in many cereals. May cause allergic reactions, interfere with elimination, and should be completely avoided in cases of coeliac disease.

INFUSION concentrated solution produced by steeping a substance in water. Often used medicinally.

INULIN natural fibre, found in artichokes, onions and garlic, that helps to moderate blood sugar levels and reduce sugar cravings, thereby reducing calorie intake.

LACTOBACILLI bacteria that are beneficial to the intestines.

LAXATIVE substance that stimulates the evacuation of faeces.

LECITHINS group of substances found in vegetables, egg yolk, milk and meat that stimulates growth and cellular nutrition.

LEVULOSE highly assimilable natural sugar, similar to glucose. Suitable for people with diabetes.

LINOLEIC AND ALPHA-LINOLEIC ACIDS essential polyunsaturated fatty acids (also known as omega-6 and omega-3 fatty acids) that are important for normal growth and development. Because they cannot be synthesized by the body they must be obtained from the diet.

MALIC ACID slightly astringent fruit acid, found in apples, that is essential for converting sugars and fats into energy.

MONOUNSATURATED FAT type of fatty acid – found in olive oil in particular – that helps prevent atherosclerosis.

OLEIC ACID monounsaturated fatty acid, found in olive oil. A high intake of oleic acid can lower cholesterol levels.

OXALATE poisonous substance found in certain plants, such as rhubarb or sorrel. Plants containing oxalate should not be eaten by those suffering from gout, arthritis or stones in the kidneys or bladder.

PAPAIN substance found in papaya that facilitates protein breakdown and aids digestion.

PECTIN water-soluble fibre – found in abundance in fruit – that has astringent properties and helps to reduce or stop diarrhoea.

PHYSALIN complex chemical found in various parts of the physalis plant. Diuretic, anti-inflammatory and helps the elimination of uric acid.

PHYTOCHEMICAL biologically-active plant compound, often of medicinal value.

POLYUNSATURATED FATS of which there are two groups: omega-3 (found in oily fish) and omega-6 fatty acids (found in vegetable oils such as sunflower or corn oil, seeds and nuts). Both are important for health.

POULTICE mixture of herbs or other substances, often heated, that is spread onto a bandage and applied to a particular body part to reduce soreness and inflammation.

QUERCETIN one of the many types of bioflavonoids, found in apples, onions and green beans. Reduces blood cholesterol levels.

RAPHANOL substance that facilitates digestion by promoting bile flow and the emptying of the gallbladder.

SATURATED FAT tends to be solid at room temperature and is found in abundance in dairy and animal fat, as well as some vegetable fat, such as palm oil. Too many saturated fats in the diet can lead to the build up of fatty deposits in the arteries.

TERPENES range of compounds, found in the essential oils of plants, that can be employed therapeutically. Should be used with care, as they may cause sensitivity reactions in some people.

TINCTURE medicinal solution in alcohol.

TONIC medicine that has an invigorating or revitalizing effect on the body.

TOPICAL TREATMENTS medical treatments that are applied directly to the affected area of skin.

TRYPTOPHAN OR L TRYPTOPHAN essential amino acid that is used by the body to build proteins and for the synthesis of the neurotransmitter serotonin. Can help to alleviate migraine and premenstrual tension.

USEFUL CONVERSIONS FROM METRIC TO IMPERIAL
25 g = 1 oz
100 g = 3½ oz
500 g = 18 oz
1 kg = 2¼ lb
25 ml = 1 fl oz
100 ml = 4 fl oz
600 ml = 20 fl oz/1 pint
1 litre = 36 fl oz

index

Bold numbers indicate a main entry in chapters one or two. For recipes using a particular food, see under the appropriate food.

bibliography

Paul Belaiche, *Traité de Phytothérapie et Aromathérapie* (Maloine S.A. Editeur, 1979)
Paul Bocuse, *La Cuisine du Marché* (Flammarion, 1976)
Arlette Braine, *Des Plantes pour Tous les Jours* (Presse Pocket, 1993)
T. Cechini, *Encyclopédie des Plantes Médicinales* (Editions De Vecchi, Paris 1993)
Anna Del Conte, *Secrets from an Italian Kitchen* (Corgi, 1989)
Marie Delmas, *Les Mille Recettes aux Mille Vertus* (Magnard/Le François, 1990)
Anne Dolamore, *Olive Oil Companion* (Macmillan, 1988)
Dorvault, *L'Officine* (23rd edition, 1995)

Duhamel, *Cahiers de Phytothérapie*, (Masson Editions, Paris)
Jeanette Ewin, *The Plants We Need to Eat* (Thorsons, 1997)
Brigitte Fichaux, *La Nouvelle Cuisine Familiale* (Les Editions Gabriandre, La Cure, 30960 St Jean de Valeriscle)
Jane Grigson, *Jane Grigson's Fruit Book* (Penguin, 1983)
Catherine Kousmine, *La Méthode Kousmine* (Editions Jouvence, 1989)
Henry Leclerc, *Précis de Phytothérapie* (Masson, 1994)
Miriam Polunin, *Healing Foods* (Dorling Kindersley, 1997)
Marie-Antoinette Mulot, *Votre Santé par les Elixirs* (Editions du

Dauphin, Paris, 1986)
Berthe Pizzigoni, *La Cuisine Végétarienne pour Tous* (Editions De Vecchi poche, 1993)
Maria Luisa Rapaggi, *Erborare e Cucinare* (Edagricole Edizioni Agricole, Bologna, 1995)
Jean Valnet, *Aromathérapie* (Maloine S.A. Editeur, 1984)
Jean Valnet, *Phytothérapie* (Maloine S.A. Editeur, 1983)
Jean Valnet, *Fruits et Legumes* (Maloine S.A. Editeur, 1985)
Various authors, *A Taste of History* (English Heritage, 1993)
Jacques Veissid, *Traité de Médecine Populaire* (Société Parisienne d'Edition, Paris, 1973)

Acknowledgments
Duncan Baird Publishers would like to thank:

Dr Damien Downing (medical consultant)
Caroline Yates (recipe consultant)
Emma Bentham-Wood (photographer's assistant)
Juss Herd (assistant food stylist)
Ingrid Lock (indexer)

With special thanks to:

Laurent and Mary Boileau (chefs) for advice on the recipes.